487

What price independence?

Independent living and people with high support needs

Ann Kestenbaum

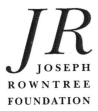
JR
JOSEPH
ROWNTREE
FOUNDATION

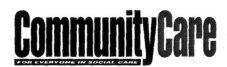
CommunityCare
FOR EVERYONE IN SOCIAL CARE

First published in Great Britain in 1999 by
The Policy Press
University of Bristol
34 Tyndall's Park Road
Bristol BS8 1PY
Telephone: +44 (0)117 954 6800
Fax: +44 (0)117 973 7308
E-mail: tpp@bristol.ac.uk
Website: http://www.bristol.ac.uk/Publications/TPP

Reprinted 2001

ISBN 1 86134 203 9

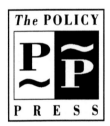

The *Community Care into Practice* series has been established by *Community Care* and the Joseph Rowntree Foundation to make research available in the social care field to a wide audience of managers and practitioners.

Community Care is the leading magazine in the field of social care. It has supported this report as part of its commitment to debate and the dissemination of information.

The report was written by **Ann Kestenbaum**, Researcher, The Disablement Income Group.

The **Joseph Rowntree Foundation** has supported this project as part of its programme of research and innovative development projects, which it hopes will be of value to policy makers and practitioners. The facts presented and views expressed in this report, however, are those of the author and not necessarily those of the Foundation.

Designed by Adkins Design
Printed and bound in Great Britain by Hobbs the Printers Ltd, Southampton

Contents

[Please note: those readers requiring an Executive Summary should refer to the summaries at the ends of Chapters 4, 5, 6, 7 and 8, and to the Conclusions, Chapter 9.]

Acknowledgements

I would like to thank all who contributed to the work that led to this report. They included staff of the Joseph Rowntree Foundation, which commissioned the research, The Disablement Income Group which hosted it, and the Independent Living Funds, which supported it. Certain individuals regularly gave their time and professional support as members of an advisory group: Jane Campbell, David Ellis, Clare Evans, Ray Jones, Alex O'Neil, Simon Stockton, Richard Tower and Helena Cava. Helena also worked with me for part of the project, carrying out many of the research interviews. Other interviewers were Marilyn Bird, Pauline Greaves and Nicola Hendey.

I also want to thank all those interviewed during the research: the social and health services staff, the voluntary sector workers and the 58 disabled people with high support needs who shared their experience with us.

1
Introduction

This report is about the situation of disabled people with high support needs. For the purpose of our research, 'high support needs' were defined in terms of the costs of community care packages, those with provision costing more than £400 a week being the main focus of our attention. In Chapter 2, the reasons for choosing that particular threshold of funding will become apparent.

The research was concerned with people, aged 18 to 70, whose primary impairments were physical and whose ability to live in the community rather than in residential care was dependent upon the policies and practices of public funding agencies, in particular local authorities (LAs), health authorities (HAs) and the Independent Living Funds (ILFs).

Beyond examining whether and how people with high support needs were being enabled to stay in the community, we were also concerned to know how satisfactorily their 'social health' needs were being met. We hoped that an exploration of the extent to which the values of independent living were being realised would provide some important insight into the factors that should be taken into account in debates about who should fund expensive care packages, also how funding and provision might be better coordinated and delivered.

There were a number of broad background questions: What *is* effective community care for severely disabled people? Is this necessarily costly? Can any costs be lowered without reducing the quality of the provision? How are expenditure limits set and how are disabled people's demands for independent living to be viewed in this context?

These are consistent with the sorts of question that the government's 'Best Value' initiative now

requires LAs to address. The Best Value approach, together with the emphasis on promoting independence advocated throughout the 1998 White Paper, *Modernising social services* (DoH, 1998), raises certain issues about services for disabled people with high support needs. These concern, on the one hand, the effective use of currently available resources and, on the other, the willingness of society to pay more in order to ensure better-quality services and more effective outcomes.

One of the consequences of constrained provider budgets has been that definitions of need now have little meaning outside the prioritisation criteria LAs construct in order to stay in budget (Davis et al, 1997). The more publicised consequences of this rationing of social care have been about hospital bed-blocking (usually applying to people waiting for residential or nursing home places), or about the loss of services by people with low-level needs because resources are targeted upon those facing crises. As this report will show, however, service reductions and tighter eligibility criteria have been affecting everyone who depends upon LA support. People with high support needs who want to stay in the community are particularly vulnerable, not only because the quality of their lives is so greatly determined by the appropriateness and quality of the services they are offered, but because they often fear rocking the boat that keeps them afloat in the community if they challenge professionals' decisions about those services.

Best Value demands an examination of the *outcomes* of community care policies and practices, but it is unlikely that these can be adequately assessed purely in terms of objective, quantitative measures. The values of independent living, emphasising as they do individual differences and disabled people's rights to choice and control in their everyday activities, do not easily lend themselves to blueprints for particular services. There cannot be a simple equating of independent living with particular practices such as direct payments, for example, or with any particular type of social activity.

By focusing upon the outcomes for people with high-level support needs, within a framework set by independent living values, we hope to have contributed towards the development of more flexible, high-quality responses to those needs, encouraging some further consideration of how current resources might be better used and how new resources such as the Social Services Modernisation Fund might be targeted.

The impetus and funding for this work came from the Joseph Rowntree Foundation and the project was led by the author of this report working with The Disablement Income Group, an organisation dedicated to improving the financial circumstances of disabled people through programmes of advice, advocacy, publications, research and training.

2

Background

Local authorities and community care

With the implementation of the 1990 NHS and Community Care Act, new arrangements for funding support for elderly and disabled people came into being. Money transferred from Social Security to local authorities (LAs) in the form of a Special Transitional Grant could be used to pay for residential places, or it could be used to fund packages of support which would enable recipients to remain in their own homes.

An initial claim, sometimes presented as the primary purpose of the legislation, was that people with high support needs would have more choice. Instead of entering residential care when their condition deteriorated, or their informal carers could no longer cope, they could be provided with a mix of domiciliary, day centre and respite services by a social services department (SSD) which, unlike Social Security, could manage this package as well as fund it.

The more powerful imperative behind the legislation - the government's determination to control escalating public expenditure on social care - has made LAs into the gatekeepers of provision which, whether residential or community care, has become ever more tightly constrained by cash limits. In this situation, the choice between residential and community provision for individuals with severe disabilities can become less a response to their need for support and ambitions for independent living than a response to cost comparisons between the two types of provision.

As early as 1994, a letter from the Department of Health, widely circulated around SSDs, warned that the community care reforms should be seen to be not about choice between residential care and community care but only about choice between different residential homes (DoH, 1994). Since

then there has been the Gloucestershire judgment, which has given LAs the right to take resources into account when offering services, and more and more indications that social services are imposing ceilings on the costs of individual packages.

In 1993/94 it was clear that at least some SSDs were prepared to use part of the community care Special Transitional Grant to cover the cost of expensive care packages (Kestenbaum, 1996). Since then, however, there have been budget cuts in the context of which individual high-cost packages can appear in stark relief against the competition of other services and client groups for the same financial resources. This may be particularly noticeable when budgets have been not only reduced, but divided between new unitary authorities (Craig, 1993). Social services have generally been targeting their resources towards people in greatest need but have been sensitive to criticisms of the 'gearing effect', that is, expenditure on high-cost packages means that people with less intense needs may get no service at all (Audit Commission, 1997).

Providers in the independent sector have observed that the impact of ceilings on support packages has been an increasing number of requests for quick visit services of 15 minutes or less, plus pressures to provide higher quality care at the same or reduced costs - "allowing minimum time for minimum service" (Hardy, 1998).

Community support *may* be cheaper than residential care, particularly where there is informal support from relatives. But some packages can be more expensive, especially if compared with the cost of basic non-specialised residential or nursing home provision. In these circumstances it may be argued that a consideration of cost-*effectiveness* as opposed to cost-*benefit* (or *efficiency*) is necessary if the principles of independent living and disabled people's rights to choice and control are to be respected. This would mean an emphasis first and foremost on the quality of the outcome that is to be desired, followed by an effort to achieve that outcome as cheaply as possible, rather than an emphasis on an amount of money made available followed by an attempt to get the most out of it.

In practice there is of course a case for both effectiveness and efficiency, and the replacement of Compulsory Competitive Tendering, in which price was paramount, by Best Value, with its emphasis on achieving higher quality outcomes throughout LA activities, will have an important impact on all social services users to the extent that both are achieved.

Other key aspects of the government's new agenda for improving social care include: the desire to drive up standards and attain greater consistency of services; the social inclusion of traditionally marginalised groups; and the development of joint working and partnership across agencies. One important statement for disabled people in the White Paper (DoH, 1998) is the following about the objectives of social services:

> ... to maximise the benefit to service users for the resources available, and to demonstrate the effectiveness and value for money of the care and support provided, and allow for choice and different responses for different needs and circumstances

Residential care and perverse incentives

A perverse financial incentive currently operates against the intended aim of community care when the net cost to a LA of a residential placement is less than the cost of supporting the person in their own home. This net cost is arrived at after recouping the social security residential allowance (£57.50 outside greater London, £64 within) and

other non-disregardable income, including the person's state pension, from the gross cost of the placement. In its 1998 White Paper, the government suggested phasing out the residential allowance and transferring resources to LAs.

For 1998/99, the rates set by the Department of Social Security (DSS) for care home residents with preserved rights (applicable to pre-1993 placements) were £213 (residential home) and £318 (nursing home) for elderly people. For younger physically disabled people they were £292 and £359 respectively.

In recent years, the baseline fees that LAs have been willing to pay for placements have tended to match the social security levels for elderly people, but there is now more evidence of them setting their own rates (sometimes lower than the DSS rate), according to a local market in which they have become a major player (Laing & Buisson Ltd, 1998a). For younger disabled people, however, authorities may have to pay considerably more than the DSS rate. One reason for this is that there has been little activity in the market for homes for this group and places are harder to find (unlike the situation for people with learning disabilities where the hospital resettlement programme provided a spur). Another is that places for under-65s often have to be negotiated individually because of specialist requirements, and they are expensive because of those requirements.

The higher costs of institutional care for those with severe physical disabilities should raise the amount LAs are willing to spend on the alternative of community care, but another development should be noted. Local authorities' power in the care home market, it is claimed, has increased the level of dependency of people admitted to dual-registered residential homes. They may in effect be "buying nursing on the cheap" (Laing & Buisson Ltd, 1998a).

The Independent Living Funds

Shortly before the implementation of the new community care legislation in 1993 came another change which was likely to have an important effect on the ability of people with high support needs to live in the community. The original Independent Living Fund (ILF), which offered financial help to severely disabled people so that, independent of LAs in many cases, they could stay in their own homes, closed its doors to new applicants.

The ILF was replaced by two new discretionary trusts, funded, like the original one, by central government: the ILF Extension Fund and the ILF 1993 Fund (usually now referred to as the 93 Fund). The Extension Fund has continued payments to established clients of the old ILF, but its cash limits have precluded inflation-linked increases in awards. No increases at all were available during its first year and after that were considered only if there had been a significant increase in care needs (though this requirement has recently been relaxed to some extent). The Extension Fund operates a £560 ceiling on its awards.

The 93 Fund was open to new applicants but has operated on a different basis from the old ILF. It offers only 'top-up' awards to disabled people aged 16 to 65 who get at least £200 worth of services from social services. This Fund thus gives LAs the opportunity to assess and then support more expensive packages of community support without spending more than £200 per week themselves, an amount meant to correspond to the average net cost to a LA of a nursing home placement. (Appendix A lists the full 93 Fund eligibility criteria and allowable uses of awards.)

However, these opportunities are constrained by a rule that limits the overall joint LA/93 Fund contribution to a care package to £500 a week, a figure which does not appear to have been based upon any particular evidence of care costs and which has remained the same since the Fund's establishment in 1993. (Packages can rise above £500 after six months if social services are willing to increase their contributions, but the 93 Fund can never pay more than £300 per week.)

For clients of the ILFs, means-tested charges have always been made. This has sometimes deterred people from wanting to apply, particularly those with working spouses, if they could get an acceptable service from their LA with lower or nil charge.

The NHS and community care

A higher profile debate is currently going on about the boundaries between health and social services responsibilities. The NHS Continuing Care guidance was published in February 1995 but provided only broad guidelines (DoH, 1995). It was left to HAs and LAs to work out detailed agreements about how responsibilities would be divided and how funding from the NHS could be used to compensate for shifts in those responsibilities. In practice, care management, which was originally meant to coordinate tailor-made packages across different agencies, including health, has offered access only to social services budgets. Although health and social services budgets may in some places have been aligned and joint commissioning managers appointed, there remains considerable scope for conflict between agencies and concern on the part of users who now have to face means-tests for services that used to be free. A report by the House of Commons Select Health Committee (1999) condemned the lack of vision of professional bodies which were perpetuating the divide at the expense of users and carers.

The government White Paper *Modernising social services* (DoH, 1998) has promised to address this major problem by legislating to make it easier for social services and health authorities (HAs) to work together through pooled budgets, lead commissioning and integrated provision. These will still be permissive powers. Possibly a more significant long-term development will be primary care groups, as described in the previous year's White Paper for Health, *The new NHS* (DoH, 1997a), but social services seem likely to have a low input into these groups. For disabled (as opposed to ill) people, there is a fear that they may *not* be a positive development if they embody a retreat to the dominance of the medical model of assessment and provision.

The Royal Commission on Long Term Care

Shortly before this report was completed, the report of the Royal Commission on Long Term Care (1999) was published, proposing that social care, like nursing care, should be provided free to all users and paid for out of general taxation. The investigation was largely concerned with the support of older people because of the numerical importance of that client group, but it was recommended that younger disabled people should be treated in the same way. Current indications are that the government will view the Commission's proposals as necessitating an unacceptably high tax burden, in which case means-tested charges on social care will continue to be imposed. In recent years, these charges by LAs have been significantly increased to help meet community care costs, creating a major problem for people with high support needs by further reducing their ability to self-fund aspects of independent living not covered by their care packages (Kestenbaum, 1997).

Direct payments

The implementation of direct payments legislation in April 1997, which enabled LAs to provide cash payments instead of services to people in the 18 to 65 age group, was intended to open up opportunities for disabled people to have more choice and flexibility.

The Department of Health is currently carrying out a review of how direct payments have been

operating. Meanwhile, the government announced in the social services White Paper (DoH, 1998) that the option of direct payment will be extended to over-65s (presumably on the same basis as for the under-65s, that LAs have the power but not the legal obligation to do so).

Previous research had suggested that direct payments could be less expensive than LA-managed services (Zarb and Nadash, 1994). In the case of ILF awards this is almost certainly true because the Funds' administration costs are less than 2% of their total budget, but the ILFs are charitable trusts without the various statutory responsibilities for assessment, provision and quality control which are attached to LAs (Independent Living Fund, 1998). Already it is clear that many LA direct payments schemes are acknowledging the add-on costs involved for people who manage their own personal assistance, and the ILF, in its contributions towards joint-funded packages, is also now willing to match rates for direct payments accepted by SSDs. Some LAs have responded to the recommendation that dedicated support systems be set up (Hasler et al, 1999). Support schemes, it is argued, can make direct payments cost-effective by replacing some care management functions.

When direct payments were made legal, social services were expected to offer an individual only that option where the cost would not exceed that of the services they replaced (DoH, 1997b). It remained to be seen whether direct payments would make expensive care packages cheaper while at the same time improving quality of outcome for the user. There has been a continuing concern, however, that, in a climate of financial constraint, social services might treat direct payments as desirable *only* because they were a cheap option and be prepared to fund them only on that basis.

3
The research

Promoting independent living for disabled people involves a much wider range of services and support than we were able to cover within the scope of this project. Housing and education, for example, are major considerations. There is also an important interface between the availability of appropriate housing and the provision of domiciliary care, and some observations about this are included in the report. Equipment is similarly an essential consideration. Our main focus, however, was upon the need for high levels of personal assistance and the question of how this is funded.

Aims

The aims of our project were threefold:

- To establish what constitutes 'high support needs' and why it is that the cost of some disabled people's community care packages are above £400 a week. This would mean identifying the needs-related factors that contribute to high costs and how local circumstances (including the policies of funding agencies), rather than just individual circumstances, affect these costs.

- To find out how expensive support packages are currently funded and describe the partnerships that operate between funding agencies such as LAs, the Independent Living Funds and HAs. Where partnerships for people with high support needs appear to promote independent living effectively, what range of options does this represent? And where independent living arrangements are unsatisfactory, what are the reasons for this?

- To explore the effect that the current regulations or budget constraints of these funding agencies are having on their

continuing abilities to support high-cost care packages. The £500 limit of the ILF 93 Fund, the imposition of ceilings on costs by LAs and the redesignation of responsibilities between social care and healthcare providers would be examined in relation to whether disabled people with high-cost support needs remain in the community with adequate support, whether they remain with *in*adequate support, or whether they are obliged to accept residential care.

Method

After consulting a range of organisations and individuals with relevant knowledge and experience, we began the first stage of the research with an examination of information available through the ILFs. This information included statistics about recipients of high-cost care packages and about applications to the 93 Fund from different LAs, which were of interest in themselves and helped in selecting a sample of authorities for the later stage of the research. The ILFs also provided a useful input of experience from office staff who processed applications, from Visiting Social Workers (VSWs) who assessed applicants and from the Funds' Contact Officers (COs) in SSDs. Study days, attended by both VSWs and COs, were held during the early months of our project and provided an opportunity to discuss issues around high support needs.

The ILFs also facilitated confidential access to case files. Through an examination of a selection of these it was possible to pursue our first aim of identifying the elements that contributed to the high costs of care packages (see Chapter 4).

The second stage of the research was an exploration of what was going on in six selected

LAs. In each case this involved interviews with staff of both statutory and voluntary sector agencies and with disabled people with high support needs. The latter were identified through a combination of the ILFs, SSDs and disabled people's organisations and were people whose care costs were above £400 a week, that is, well above the basic costs of residential and nursing home placements and approaching the joint funding limit imposed by the 93 Fund.

The reason for spreading our investigation over six different authorities was not to make direct comparisons between them, but to achieve a range of different contexts in which to identify and examine relevant issues. In choosing the authorities we had to bear this in mind while ensuring that there would be enough people with high support needs available to interview.

In total, there were interviews with 50 people from LAs and HAs (including senior strategic and operational managers and front-line social workers/care managers) and 12 people from voluntary organisations (including several that ran direct payment support schemes). In each case the objective was to gather information about structures and policies and to explore different perspectives on the following: access to and range of services provided; flexibility of services; decisions about funding; National Health Service (NHS) input to community care; use of the ILFs; involvement of the voluntary sector; direct and indirect payments; charging policies; and other local issues raised in the course of the research.

We interviewed 58 disabled service users (between 7 and 12 per authority). These semi-structured interviews were carried out by a total of four research assistants working for the project and were designed to elicit information about the person's current support arrangements, how and why they developed as they did, and how satisfactory they were. People were encouraged to

think about what worked well for them, but also about any compromises or sacrifices they were forced to make. Most interviews lasted for about 90 minutes.

Table 1 provides some age, gender and household information about the disabled people interviewed in the six authorities and Appendix B provides a brief description of each person referred to, or quoted, in the report.

Table 1: Disabled interviewees - characteristics

Age	
21-30	10
31-40	19
41-50	17
51-60	9
61-70	3
Total	*58*
Gender	
Male	22
Female	36
Total	*58*
Household	
Alone	29
With spouse/partner	14
With parent(s)	10
With other	1
Single parent	2
Residential care	2
Total	*58*

The six authorities

The six authorities were all in England: two in the North (Authorities B and C), three in the Midlands (A, D and F) and one in London (E). Authority A was a rural authority and F was a new unitary. They had numbers of ILF 93 Fund clients ranging from 6.5 to 24.9 per 100,000 population (England average 6.4) and of ILF Extension Fund

Table 2: Disabled interviewees - funding sources

Authority	Total no	Funding source							
		LA only	LA + 93F	LA + ExF	LA + HA	LA + 93F + HA	LA + ExF + HA	ExF	Res care
A	11	4	4	2	-	-	-	-	1
B	9	1	6	1	-	-	-	1	-
C	7	-	3	-	2	1	-	-	1
D	10	1	3	3	-	2	1	-	-
E	12	3	7	1	1	-	-	-	-
F	9	2	5	1	1	-	-	-	-
Total	*58*	*11*	*28*	*8*	*4*	*3*	*1*	*1*	*2*

LA = local authority; 93F = ILF 93 Fund; EXF = ILF Extension Fund; HA = health authority

clients ranging from 16.5 to 41.0 per 100,000 population (England average 15.5).

They represented a range of different stages in terms of developing indirect or direct payments schemes, including one with a very small number of long established direct payments recipients only, one with an indirect payments scheme which had not worked very well, and one with a rapidly growing direct payments scheme.

Three of the SSDs had separate physical disability teams and three operated teams that covered services for both younger physically disabled and elderly people.

Table 2 provides information about social care funding for our disabled interviewees in each authority.

4
High-cost packages

Numbers of disabled people with high-cost packages

It is difficult to find out exactly how many high-cost community care packages are currently funded by social services departments (SSDs). The main reason for this is that funding may come from several different budgets within a department. If care packages are supported solely from the Special Transitional Grant and/or the department has a well-developed financial monitoring system, then the full costs of individual packages may be known but, particularly if in-house services such as Homecare and day centres are involved, total inputs may not be costed on an individual basis and statistics not held in an accessible form.

A survey of SSDs carried out by the ILFs in 1997 asked whether they were supporting people in the community whose social care (ie domiciliary care, day centre provision and respite care) cost the authority more than £500 a week. The response from 80 authorities indicated that numbers were low but variable. Four authorities supported more than 30 packages, but more than a quarter were not supporting anyone costing more than £500; 14 authorities were unable to quantify an answer to the question for under-65s, 26 for over-65s.

Overall numbers for high-cost community care packages funded solely by social services may be difficult to ascertain, but it is possible to know about the full individual costs of those packages that are supported by the ILF 93 Fund. This is because a SSD has to demonstrate the value of its own input at a level of at least £200 worth of services a week in order to prove that it meets the Fund's eligibility criteria. Data from the ILFs made available to our research showed that, by December 1998, the ILF 93 Fund was supporting a total of 3,213 disabled people where the joint

ILF/LA contribution was more than £400 a week. In 537 of these, it was more than £500 a week. (Although the 93 Fund's maximum contribution remains £300 per week, its £500 joint contribution limit applies only to the first six months of a jointly funded package.) Table 3 shows more detail.

Table 3: Numbers of high-cost ILF 93 Fund clients	
93 Fund plus SSD combined funding (£ per week)	Number of clients (%)
More than £400	3,213 (67)
More than £450	2,209 (46)
More than £500	537 (11)
More than £550	248 (5)
More than £600	136 (3)
More than £650	92 (2)
More than £700	63 (1)
All awards	4,794 (100)
Source: ILF 93 Fund, December 1998	

It is important to note that the *full* cost of these care packages, as opposed to the 'net public purse' cost represented by the ILF/LA contribution, would include the disabled person's own financial contribution by way of ILF and LA charges. On average, clients getting more than £400 from the ILF and their LA contribute an additional £43 towards their care. Those getting more than £500 contribute on average £48.

It was also possible to get data from the ILF Extension Fund about its more expensive individual care packages but, because there is no requirement by this Fund that there must first be a contribution from the LA, its database records do not contain detail of any social services input (though this information is currently being collected through the Fund's revisit programme). We do know, however, that by December 1998 the Extension Fund was contributing more than £400 a week to 651 clients and more than £500 a week to 204 of these. Many of these disabled people would also be making a personal financial contribution to their care costs and some would have some additional social services input. Table 4 provides more detail of Extension Fund awards.

The numbers cited above for both ILF 93 Fund and Extension Fund clients do not take into account any social care funding by *health* authorities. In July 1997, an examination of case files of 95 of the 104 clients who were at that time getting the 93 Fund's maximum award of £300 revealed that seven of them were getting a financial contribution to their care package from their HA in addition to the ILF/LA input. These contributions varied from £50 to £537 a week. This would be additional to any direct provision from the district nurse service. Chapter 7 will later show the importance of the fact that the 93 Fund ignores any NHS contribution towards care packages for the purpose of its £500 limit, even if that money is channelled through social services.

Table 4: Numbers of high-cost ILF Extension Fund clients

Extension Fund award (£ per week)	Number of clients (%)
More than £400	651 (6)
More than £450	412 (4)
More than £500	204 (2)
More than £550	93 (1)
More than £600	1 (-)
All awards	10,439 (100)

Source: ILF Extension Fund, December 1998

(Note that this does not apply to NHS 'dowries' in the case of long-stay hospital closures.)

An analysis of the households of the clients getting the highest 93 Fund awards in July 1997 revealed that 45% of these were to people who lived alone. It also revealed that, in 20 of the 95 cases, clients had agreed to pay more than their assessed contribution towards their care costs in order to be eligible for the Fund's help by keeping the public purse total below £500. In some cases this extra was less than £1 a week; in others it was as much as £80. Unless paid by a relative or someone else, the additional contribution would have come from income or savings that were at or below Income Support levels. After six months, social services could pick up this extra cost, but there was no clear evidence in the ILF files as to how often this happened. Where the Fund is already contributing its maximum £300, it does not comprehensively record subsequent increases in social services input because these do not have a direct bearing on its own payments. An important consequence of this is that the figures in Table 3 should be treated as *minima*.

The percentages of high-cost 93 Fund clients in the six authorities covered during our research confirm and illustrate the uneven spread of high-level funding and indicate significant differences in social services policies or practices (see Table 5). The *total* number of 93 Fund clients in these authorities was 354.

The total number of Extension Fund clients in the six authorities was 698. Overall, just 2% of these had an award of more than £500, but this percentage varied from 0 to 15 in the different authorities, a variation likely to be a result of a number of factors affecting applications to the original ILF between 1988 and 1993.

Table 5: High-cost ILF 93 Fund clients in the six authorities (December 1998)

Local authority	Percentage of 93 Fund clients jointly funded above £500	Percentage of 93 Fund clients getting more than £300 from social services
A	31	4
B	22	8
C	33	18
D	31	4
E	61	39
F	48	0
Overall	34	10

Source: ILF 93 Fund, December 1998

Use of the ILFs

The numbers of ILF 93 Fund clients in each of the six authorities of our study varied considerably, there clearly being a much higher culture of ILF use in some areas than in others. Changes have sometimes come about as a result of deliberate take-up campaigns by SSDs and new direct payments schemes.

Managers and social workers in the SSDs we visited made a range of comments about use of the Funds in their authorities (some of these are expanded upon in later sections of the report):

- Many social workers are still not fully aware of the potential offered by the ILF for enhancing the care packages of some of their high support clients. Sometimes, that awareness and expertise in making application to the Fund reside in a small number of staff, often those with a current or residual specialist disability role. Others can be influenced by adverse comments about the time taken to deal with the paperwork, the time taken to get an award successfully negotiated, or bad experiences of care packages collapsing.

- The length of time it takes to process applications to the Fund can be a problem in cases where arrangements have to be put into place urgently. Apart from these crisis management problems, people have to be in receipt of the highest-rate care component of the Disability Living Allowance (DLA) and social workers complained that they did not have the time to challenge negative DLA decisions through appeals. Some also observed that it was becoming more difficult to get people onto the higher rate.

- It can be easier to get awards for people with high support needs who have learning difficulties than for people with only physical disabilities, because the former are more likely to use day centres. The cost of day centre provision contributes towards the 93 Fund threshold and may account for the full £200 if the placement is five days at £40 a day, say. The Fund has been willing to pay for an assistant to accompany a client at a day centre where one-to-one attention is required and the person would not otherwise be able to attend, but it has to be convinced that the extra care needed is not a consequence of LA staff cuts and it has refused some applications on these grounds.

- There is a particular concern about applying for the maximum 93 Fund award for an individual when there is little likelihood of social services being able to raise their contribution when either support needs or rates of pay increase. There is also a general concern that ILF awards are not automatically increased to cover normal inflationary rises in costs and the Fund cannot even consider any increase if the award is at the maximum level. Dedicated privately employed personal assistants may be prepared to keep their wages down but agencies are not, and social services have found themselves bearing the extra costs of 'ILF hours'.

- Where the 93 Fund has been contributing less than its maximum but care needs have increased, the Fund has typically expected social services to share any increase on a 50/50 basis, but recently, with less pressure on its own budget, it has been prepared to pay more where a SSD is up against rigid limits of its own and residential care has been the only alternative for the person concerned.

- The ILF has made it possible to empty whole residential care units by helping to make community care packages viable. But the time it takes to get an ILF application processed and the award confirmed can sometimes make it very difficult for someone moving out of residential care or hospital, especially where housing arrangements need coordination.

- LA packages are often rejigged to ensure eligibility for the ILF. For example, social services will substitute some respite care instead of domiciliary provision knowing that the ILF will cover the latter but not the former.

- Apart from cases where the total cost could not be contained within £500, there were circumstances where the ILF might be thought inappropriate, for example, where a partner's income would be taken into account by the ILF but not by the LA, or where a partner refused to declare their income. If an authority imposed lower charges than the ILF, then a disabled person might well prefer to have social services direct payments or even direct provision rather than means-tested ILF help.

- Some social workers regretted the loss of the original ILF because the change had forced some people to accept help from social services when they would have preferred not to and curtailed opportunities that had once existed for creative packages

Other sources of funding

Social security provides the main source of finance with which the majority of severely disabled people support their independence in the community. Apart from DLA, which was available to everyone in our sample on the grounds of their high support needs, there was also the Severe Disablement Premium (payable to those who lived alone with nobody claiming Invalid Care Allowance for providing assistance) and various transitional and preserved rights dating from earlier social security arrangements. It was in the interests of social services to ensure that these benefits were maximised.

Another important source of financial support for some people comes from compensation awards. There can be a major cultural difference between the circumstances of people who have compensation awards and those with congenital impairments who are dependent on Income Support, but the former are not excluded from LA help and not even from ILF help. If money is tied up in a trust in such a way that the disabled person does not have access to it to pay for everyday social care and their accessible capital is less than £8,000, then they might still be eligible for an ILF award. The difference tends to show up in the quality of their housing and equipment. At least one SSD in our research was making efforts to tighten up their eligibility criteria and charging systems in relation to people receiving compensation payments.

Factors contributing to high costs

The primary objective of the 1997 examination of ILF 93 Fund case files carried out in an early stage of this research was to identify a range of factors which contributed to particularly high care costs. This, together with observations from ILF staff who are familiar with the full range of clients, suggested the following needs-related circumstances (as opposed to local policies or care management practice) that could be seen to contribute to the high cost of care packages:

- *The disabled person is living alone with little or no informal care.* Sometimes disabled people have moved out of institutional care into independent living in adapted properties. Sometimes they are committed to remaining in their own home after an informal carer (usually parent or spouse) has left or died. Alternatively they have lived alone for some time but their condition has deteriorated and their need for assistance has either suddenly or gradually increased. The absence of supportive relatives and/or friends means that there is no option but to pay for all necessary assistance. However, it is not just support packages covering 24 hours that cost more than £500 a week.

- *The disabled person is living with a parent or spouse who is unable, because of age, poor health, disability or other responsibilities (eg for children), to provide much assistance.* The availability of some informal care will reduce the cost to the LA/ILF, but sometimes not by enough to keep it below £500. Of the 95 cases with costs over £500, 21 were disabled people living with a parent or partner.

- *Night-time cover is necessary.* The cost of having assistance available at night varies considerably, from the relatively cheap cost of a night-time alarm system, through to having someone sleeping over who is likely to be called upon only occasionally, to having active night care where the cost is calculated on the basis of hourly rates. A waking night would often cost above £50 and more at weekends. To keep costs down, often some sort of 'package deal' is negotiated with an agency when night-time assistance is involved.

- *Live-in care is not appropriate.* Where a significant amount of day-time assistance is needed and night-time cover is also necessary, the cheapest option might be a live-in arrangement costing less than £500 from many agencies. This may not be appropriate, however: (a) if the assistance required is very demanding; (b) if the accommodation is unsuitable; (c) if the disabled person's desire for privacy is too heavily compromised; or (d) if the location leads to difficulties in getting a live-in assistant. Non-live-in rotas of agency workers which cover the full 24 hours are usually much more expensive, with higher rates for unsocial hours in evenings and at weekends and bank holidays.

- *Travel costs of assistants are high because of rural isolation.* Not only the travel costs themselves but the extra time spent travelling are significant. This also applies to transport to day centres and other activities.

- *Appropriate day centre provision is available only if an extra person is available to provide one-to-one assistance.* Increasingly, day centres have been unable to offer the extra staff time sometimes needed.

- *Two assistants are needed frequently for moving and handling.* Recent health and safety rules for social services and agency staff have had a significant impact.

- *Two or more assistants are needed for certain tasks when there are severe behavioural problems.*

- *Highly trained assistants are needed because of special feeding or handling requirements.*

- *A high level of domestic cleaning is needed because of the risk of infection.*

- *Because of risk, eg fits, risk of choking or behaviour problems, 24-hour care/supervision is necessary.* The ILF will fund supervision only where there is an ever-present risk rather than when it is just general encouragement that is required.

Some of the factors associated with behavioural problems and the need for 24-hour supervision because the person is at constant risk are particularly relevant for people with a cognitive impairment. Just over one third of the Fund's maximum awards were to these clients. In general, packages for people with complex disabilities that include a cognitive impairment are feasible for under £500 only when there is an unpaid input from informal carers, usually parents, but also sometimes when accommodation is shared with others with similar needs so that provision such as night-time cover can be shared.

Summary

The ILFs are involved in supporting more than 4,000 social care packages costing above £400 a week. Apart from these, it is difficult to know exactly how many more are funded by LAs alone, because many authorities do not record the total costs of individual packages where components such as in-house homecare or day centre provision are accounted for under separate budgets. There are small numbers where people get an NHS contribution towards non-nursing elements of community care packages.

However, there is clearly an uneven spread of high-level funding by social services and considerable differences in policies and practices. This includes their use of the ILF, the 93 Fund being accessed much more by some authorities than others. Various factors ranging from different perceptions of the restrictiveness of the Fund's rules and regulations to a lack of knowledge on the part of social workers appear to account for this.

A number of factors can be identified which contribute to the high costs of care packages. The number of hours required, the number of assistants needed at any one time, the cost of those assistants and the feasibility of live-in help are affected not only by people's impairments and health, but also by their housing and location, the availability of informal unpaid care and, more recently, by policies such as lifting restrictions.

5
Budget constraints

Pressures on social services budgets

Five of the six LAs covered by our research had recently experienced pressures on their social services budgets, which had a significant impact upon expenditure on people with high support needs. The sixth authority was anticipating such an impact the following year. Some care managers observed that the effect on users was being exacerbated by a simultaneous squeeze on welfare benefits. In particular, the higher rate of DLA was being refused to people who might a year ago have expected to be awarded it.

The consequences of social services constraints relevant to our research varied from area to area, but included contractions in services and waiting lists for equipment, the prioritisation of assessment over ongoing support and review to the extent that in some cases the latter did not happen, and the imposition of ceilings on the costs of community care packages.

Half of the departments had set up panels to ration expenditure from Special Transitional Grant (STG) budgets. Decisions about high-cost packages in the rest had to be authorised by the budget-holding manager or by a senior manager. In one of the two authorities where special panels operated for under-65s, the panel had until two years ago been open to individual disabled people who wanted to put their own case. This 'enabling panel' had changed, however, as decisions had become more resource and crisis driven. Care managers for physically disabled people now had to get panel authority for *all* care packages. This put some of their clients at a disadvantage because the concentration of resources on crisis management had led to a bias towards providing for people who were hospital 'bed-blockers' or had challenging behaviour and against providing for the assistance that physically disabled people

needed for independent living. This view on the part of SSD staff who were physical disability specialists was most strongly articulated in Authorities A and C but was echoed elsewhere. The tension set up by the need to divide diminishing resources between large numbers of over-65s and comparatively small numbers of under-65s is illustrated by a comment made to the ILF by an SSD team manager:

> "Where a person with physical disabilities wishes to live alone and is having £200 from [name of LA] and £300 from the ILF, but the package is costed above £500 a week.... The issue is one of equity. I have 55 people on the waiting list for residential and nursing homecare, all over 65 years of age. How can I justify spending more than £200 a week on one person when those needing residential care will cost the LA £130 to £200 net a week? This issue of rationing resources really means asking the ILF to fund more than £300 a week."

In most of the authorities we were working in, there were small numbers of cases where disabled people had high-cost independent living packages which had been negotiated some years ago. These were being honoured, but the chances of new packages at similar levels being agreed in the present climate had drastically declined.

Contractions in services

In authority A, four members of staff had recently been made redundant in one of the two day centres for younger people with physical disabilities. This meant that some people with high support needs were unable to attend because the remaining staff were unable to offer the level of attention they required. There was no automatic substitution of any extra personal assistance at home to compensate for this. In addition some people faced the possibility of losing their ILF award because the social services input would fall below £200. Authority C had also had recent cuts leading to day centre closures and reviews of provision which cut the number of days for most users. Care managers here voiced their fears that the decrease in relief for carers and in stimulation for users was stacking up greater problems and demand in the future.

The contraction in the provision of domestic cleaning as a consequence of changes in the size and nature of in-house services, together with policies which restricted its funding through commercial agencies, was also a concern. Care managers tried to "slip it in somewhere in the care package" but were finding this increasingly difficult as the 'short visit' scenario referred to in Chapter 2 became more common.

Another important consequence of the pressures on social services for people with high support needs was, in some cases, the lack of ongoing support. One manager described what she saw as her department's emphasis on "throughput of the elderly". Long-term support for physically disabled people was not, she felt, handled well because it was not acknowledged in quantifiable work-level targets.

> "Where disabled people have no allocated social worker and are left to ring up the duty officer when there's a problem, they are likely to think 'I won't bother. I can't go through it again.' It's the less able ones who suffer from that. The able ones will cope."

We found in our research that ongoing care management support for those with high-level needs was very variable, with strong and consistent support in some cases, but inadequate contact in others (see Chapter 8).

A third general concern expressed across the board by social workers was that budget constraints led to the prioritisation of crisis management at the expense of preventative domiciliary support. As a result, the management of support for people who go on to develop high support needs was being undermined, constituting a short-sighted perspective on resource management.

Expenditure ceilings on community care packages

All six authorities imposed ceilings on the cost of community care packages. These were set with reference to (a) the cost of residential/nursing homecare, and (b) the ILF threshold. In general, ceilings were imposed more rigidly for people over 65 than for those under 65.

In Authority A, there was a wide range of residential homes in the area offering places at the Income Support rate, and the LA ceiling for over-65s was set at £100. The ceiling for under-65s with physical disabilities was £225, which became a net figure of £200 once the maximum £25 charge to the user was deducted. There had been strong pressure from within the department for the limits to be equalised at the level of £100 for all users, but this had been successfully resisted by managers for younger disabled people who drew attention to the fact that any ILF contribution would be sacrificed if the SSD ceiling was below £200. In this authority, care managers would direct cases involving people with brain injuries or complex disabilities towards the learning disability team, even if their impairments were primarily physical, because there a higher ceiling of £250 was applied.

Authority F operated a 'normal limits' policy, meaning that no more than the gross cost of appropriate residential or nursing homecare would normally be spent on a community care package. Exceptions, across the *full* age range, were subject to authorisation by the lead officer. The normal limit for someone assessed at Residential Band 5 (younger disabled person or, since 1998, very dependent older person) would be £285. At Nursing Band 1 (basic nursing) it would be £311 and at Nursing Band 3 (very highly dependent nursing care) it would be £380. The five residential bands and three nursing bands caused some difficulties because the guidelines on fitting people into them were vague. There was also an issue about how bandings matched registration categories, for example, did Band 5 link to a home actually registered for younger people with physical disabilities? One team manager suggested that in practice, for younger disabled people, sticking to 'normal limits' was more likely to be argued when someone wanted to come out of residential care than when they were at threat of having to enter it.

In Authority D, there was technically still no ceiling on community care packages but, because of a budget crisis, expenditure from the STG budget was being linked to the average cost of residential or nursing homecare. In a committee paper in late 1998, it was noted that, if formal ceilings were to be set at the *net* cost of such placements, this would be £123 for the lower level of dependency and £143 for the higher level. Instead, it was proposed that the ILF 93 Fund threshold of £200 be applied. It was thought that a future direct payments scheme could reduce the cost of some of those who currently had more expensive packages.

In Authority E, there was a rigid ceiling of £190 for people over 65 and a less rigid ceiling of £225 for under-65s. For the latter it was acknowledged that, in reality, appropriate residential placements for severely disabled younger people would have to be outside the authority, at some distance from family and friends and at an average cost of £600.

The remaining two authorities technically had no ceiling for under-65s, but in practice they both operated at the £200 ILF threshold. For over-65s the ceilings were £247 and £250, respectively.

The operation of discretion

As indicated above, although ceilings had in principle been set, discretion was more likely to be applied to decisions about funding community care for under-65s than for over-65s. Among the reasons given were that: appropriate residential care might cost a great deal more; the consequences for splitting families might be unacceptable; no appropriate local residential provision was available; and younger disabled people had a greater moral claim to independent living in the community even if this was the more expensive option. None of these arguments was universally promoted, opinions varying as to what type of residential placements were considered appropriate and the extent to which younger disabled people were entitled to levels and types of service that over-65s could not access.

In general, there were four situations where discretion might be applied in order to keep people with high support needs in the community.

● *The cost of an SSD/ILF jointly funded package which had originally been contained within £500 was now unavoidably going to cost more, but the ILF was already contributing its maximum £300 per week*

In the words of one manager in authority A, where a £200 limit was rigidly imposed:

> *"Is it right to set someone up with a £500 package when you know that they're going to deteriorate but won't get any more? Should you pitch the package at £400 initially so that you've got something to play with?"*

In practice, these questions became: 'Should *any* attempt be made to keep this person in the community?' In this authority, and probably also in the others, static conditions were more likely to get funding. This recent resource-led development meant that people with deteriorating conditions were expected to enter residential care earlier and were deprived of time they might otherwise have spent in the community. But 'pitching the package at £400 initially' would have meant constructing a care package that left a great deal to be desired in terms of risk and quality of life (see Chapter 8).

In Authority C, where a rigid ceiling applied, efforts were made to get people with deteriorating conditions onto ILF funding as early as possible, well before the need for £500 was approached. This was the case with individual social workers everywhere who had substantial experience of working with the ILF, but by no means did it extend to all social workers who worked with younger disabled people. Perhaps equally important was the ability to mobilise discretion in order to get provision 'by hook or by crook' above the £200 threshold before a crisis made it impossible to contain the package within £500. Even some of those familiar with applications to the ILF did not know that the £500 ceiling operated by the Fund applies for only six months. Although the Fund cannot then increase its contribution above £300, the LA can, if it chooses, raise its own contribution to any level it likes. Some social workers wrongly thought that such an increase would threaten all ILF input.

In practice, in Authority C, when the research was being carried out, the disability panel had only £300 of new money each week to allocate and 10 to 15 new cases being presented to it each week. In some cases, just £10 a week was being added to build a package up gradually to what was really

needed. So the leeway for any sort of discretion was very constrained.

An example from ILF files of a support package increasing to well above £500 was **Richard**:

Richard was 25 and had Friedreich's ataxia. His initial package had to be significantly increased when he had a stroke resulting in the need for very intensive help, including two people to lift him, regular assistance with toileting and feeding and also help through the night. His elderly parents could no longer provide the unpaid help they had previously provided. His total package became £650.16 for 94.5 day hours from social services and £300 for active night care plus 7 day hours from the ILF, a total cost of £950 a week.

- *A new package was going to cost more than £500 to begin with, so application for help to the ILF was not an option*

The incentive for keeping costs below £500 was considerable, but it was not always possible and in these cases there was often criticism of the ILF 93 Fund for not being prepared to operate the £300 limit on its own contribution but relax the overall £500 limit. Instead of paying, say, £250 or £300 towards a package, social services were faced with having to pay the full £550 or £600 (or insist upon a cheaper residential option).

Mark was an example of this. After a car accident, he lived alone in an extensively adapted house of his own. He had no movement except in his head and one shoulder, but was able to control an electric wheelchair. He needed someone to help him with all personal care tasks, also to cough and lean forward every hour to relieve the pressure. Transferring required two assistants and someone needed to be with him at night. A district nurse visited each morning, but the rest of his support package cost well over £500. An application to the ILF had thus failed but social services used its discretion to cover the full cost.

- *The disabled person was assessed as needing more than the SSD ceiling but was ineligible for ILF help because they failed to meet one of its criteria (ie receipt of the higher-level care component of DLA; being under 66; having income or capital below ILF limits; and having a prognosis of more than six months' life expectancy)*

The case was described of a man of 58 with muscular dystrophy who was receiving only the middle-rate care component of DLA but whose condition had deteriorated. The authority was unwilling to cover the extra cost of keeping him at home while the higher rate, which would open the way to ILF funding, was applied for. Instead he went into a nursing home where, according to his care manager, "He died a month later because he'd just given up". Two years ago, she claimed, the authority would have provided bridging funds.

- *The ILF's rule that a partner's income above Income Support level be contributed towards costs means that the disabled person is unwilling or unable to agree to an application being made*

Kirsten lived with her husband and two young children. She had multiple sclerosis and needed assistance from her husband for turning every few hours during the night. Her day-time support entailed a combination of district nurse and independent sector agency input, the latter, together with regular respite provision, costing over £400 a week. Kirsten's husband had a job and threatened to leave rather than declare his income, in which case Kirsten would not be able to keep her children. The ILF could not therefore be accessed and social services were having to fund the whole package.

Consequences of expenditure ceilings

Rigid ceilings meant that there were younger disabled people in nursing homes who did not wish to be there. The most vulnerable in this respect were single people without informal carers, people who were temporarily ill and could not, because of their illness, maintain the organisation of their care packages, and people who were not eligible for the ILF because of income or prognosis. The need for night-time provision was often the trigger for residential care to be considered.

Until two years ago in Authority C, there had been only one residential home for under-65s. This cost £520. The authority had therefore been willing to pay up to that amount for alternative community care. Now there were three new Younger Disabled Units (YDUs) which cost under £500 a place and arguing for a £500 package had become much more difficult, even though the YDUs were considered by care managers to offer an inadequate service in terms of fulfilling social needs. In some other authorities, cheaper nursing homes catering primarily for elderly people were being used for people under 65.

In Authority D, there were two residential homes for younger people which cost £565 and £603. These were considered 'reasonable', but places there were hard to get. The social workers we interviewed considered other nursing homes costing £360 to be totally inappropriate, but it was feared that the increasing pressure on funding would soon lead to their use.

In Authority E, the only acceptable residential homes were outside the area and cost more than £600. Although the nominal ceiling for care packages was £225, it was claimed that no younger disabled people had yet gone into residential care because of cost comparisons.

In Authority A, it used to be possible to set up a package costing £500, but nowadays this was unlikely. In Authority B, although there was a small number of long-established packages above £500, no new packages costing more than £500 had been submitted to the panel in the previous 18 months. The suggestion here was not that people with high support needs were going into residential care but that they were making do with less, or had been able to reduce costs by using direct payments to pay for personal assistants (see Chapter 8).

Clearly, in some places at least, care packages had been contained within £500 by lowering expectations. With certain exceptions, proposals for high-cost packages no longer reached panels or lead officers until they had been pared down to the minimum commensurate with risk assessment. Major adjustments were sometimes being made to reduce demand on the STG budget or to enable people to qualify for ILF help. Cheaper providers were sought and negotiations with agencies that were in sharp competition with each other for LA contracts were carried out.

There must clearly be a question mark over the extent to which these pared-down care packages were appropriate and satisfactory.

> *"The limit of £500, because it is so low, causes conflict between social services and ourselves as we have to get involved in so many situations where disabled people are unhappy with their care package because it is inadequate. It also demoralises social workers who feel they cannot do a good job within the financial constraints placed upon them." (Manager - local disabled people's organisation)*

The following six cases illustrate these concerns:

Pauline changed to a more expensive agency and, even though her multiple sclerosis had deteriorated, she was having to make do with five fewer hours. She was worried by her social worker's warning that there would be no additional funding available in the future.

> *"It puzzles me why they think I need two hours in the morning through the week, but they only allocate an hour and a half at the weekend. It's a bit of a push. I think it comes down to finance really because the hourly rates of the agency are higher at the weekend.... Things are a bit tight, especially at bedtime. Three quarters of an hour is not long enough to get me organised and into bed ... I think because they [the second agency] wanted to take the care package over, they tried to make their bid as competitive as possible. To do that they cut down the time they thought I would need at teatime and at bedtime, the theory being that as the carers got more used to putting me to bed they would get a bit quicker. But in practice that doesn't work out because I can only go as fast as I can go.... Social services wouldn't pay for the extra time that's actually taken, so we've got this situation where the women who come to put me to bed only get paid for three quarters of an hour even though it takes them an hour or longer. I think that's unfair."*

Tracey had spent much of her life in residential care until three years ago when social services and the ILF 93 Fund agreed a joint package of funding which enabled her to move out. This move was successful and Tracey was happy with the arrangements for 20 agency hours a day, which included night cover. Unfortunately, that agency later decided to drastically increase their costs, asking for more than £700. Social services were unwilling to raise their input and argued that, in any case, Tracey's night-time needs were really a health service responsibility. There seemed to be no guarantee of any sort of night-time attention from either health or social services. Eventually a new package was agreed with the ILF for 16 hours a day which would involve a cheaper agency and cost within the £500 limit. Tracey, who was upset at the breakdown of the package and fearful about having to return to residential care, was not happy with the new arrangement and was refusing to cooperate with social services, which she distrusted, and with the agency workers, whom she saw as trying to control her. Her refusal to compromise meant that she was currently accepting only a minimal four and a half hours a day. The idea of direct payments had been suggested to her but her isolation and distrust made her afraid:

> *"I would like something different but I'm too afraid because I don't want it worse."*

Doreen was in a nursing home for two years after an accident and was very happy to be back in the community with a support package funded with direct payments, but she sometimes found it difficult coping within the money available:

> *"I would feel a lot more comfortable, a lot more happy, a lot more safe, if there was somebody here more often. But the funding doesn't allow for it.... I have good phases and bad phases and at the moment I'm in a good phase and I'm managing. But when I've not been well it's been hard. There's three hours that nobody's there, and needing help to go to the bathroom, trying to get comfy - those silly things that most people take for granted.... You're constantly having to work within the budget, which I don't mind, but it would be nice if there was some leeway."*

Joe, who had pre-senile dementia and challenging behaviour, went into residential care costing £240 a week because his wife could no longer cope. An ideal community care package was costed at £800 (offering five days at a day centre, seven nights' sleepover, and some respite). He recently came out again at his wife's request with a cheaper package which allowed only three nights' cover.

Both **Helen** and **Laura** in Authority D were having to make do with fewer than assessed hours in order to qualify for ILF help. Helen was getting 13.5 hours a day during the week but only four hours a day at weekends and was having to rely on help from parents, neither of whom was in good health, for the missing hours. Laura, who had been assessed as needing 24-hour care, was getting seven nights but only 33 day hours.

Other examples of efforts to create or maintain support packages within SSD or ILF ceilings are given in later chapters to illustrate particular issues.

Care package funding from different budgets

In accepting any application, the ILF requires that the hours and unit costs of the SSD contribution of domiciliary care, day centre provision and regular respite be costed (other input such as social worker time and equipment is not included). The purpose of this requirement is to ascertain that the SSD is contributing at least £200 a week and that the joint package will not exceed £500. Where in-house homecare or day centre placements are involved in a jointly funded SSD/ILF package, therefore, the unit costs of these services must be provided. For care packages that do *not* involve the ILF, however, the cost of any directly provided in-house service does not always count when the ceilings discussed earlier in this chapter are imposed. Ceilings may apply only to the STG budget, the provision of in-house services being negotiated separately from other budgets.

An important consequence of this in four of the authorities visited was that there was a strong incentive for care managers to use in-house services. In authority A, for example, it was much easier for a care manager to get a 24-hour care package agreed if a significant part of it was day centre provision because this element of the package did not have to be authorised by the panel managing the community care budget. The same would have applied to in-house homecare, which until recently had been available for under-65s but was now almost exclusively used for elderly people. In some other authorities, cost ceilings meant that there was still a strong incentive to use in-house homecare to the maximum. One consequence of this could be cumbersome mixtures of in-house services and agency provision that left users with little real choice or control (see Chapter 6).

In four of our six authorities, there was a policy requirement upon all social workers to use the in-house service unless it was unable to provide the hours required. This requirement was treated with considerable variation, even by social workers within the same authority and particularly by those who worked with younger disabled people (see Chapter 6).

Where in-house services were costed within care packages, for ILF or other purposes, the unit costs used showed that they were not the cheapest option, so there must have been other reasons, such as those described above, for using them. (Other research has indicated that in-house homecare may be as much as 80% more expensive than private sector provision; Laing & Buisson, 1998a.)

In Authority D, it was claimed that the unit costs of in-house homecare fell between the higher cost of voluntary sector agencies and the lower cost of the private sector. Current budget constraints meant that the voluntary sector agencies which had previously been favoured were now having to justify in detail their higher prices.

Another important incentive for promoting day centre provision, other than minimising the elements of funding that had to be secured via a panel from the community care budget, has been mentioned before. This was that it was the simplest way to lift the SSD input to the £200 threshold required by the ILF. Five days of day centre provision might well be costed at or above that target, meaning that more flexible funding of, for example, night care or weekend care through ILF direct payment could then become available. In practice this option was often blocked by the lack of day centre facilities that younger disabled people would consider acceptable.

Charging

A consequence of social services budget constraints across the board has been the introduction of charges to service users, regimes varying widely around the country (Bennett, 1996). In our research, most of the disabled people interviewed were paying a level of charge that they found acceptable, but it should be noted that the charging regimes in these authorities were less stringent than in many other areas. The charges made to people in our research were generally equal to, or less than, those operated by the ILF. (Note that, for any new application, the ILF reduces its charge by an amount equal to that levied by social services, but it will not increase any *established* award to cover a shortfall caused by *new* LA charges.)

In Authority A, people getting DLA paid a maximum of £25 a week. In B, the maximum payable was £45, but banded below that according to receipt of Income Support and DLA, and there was no charge for people on direct payments. There was a maximum of £21.50 in C, £20.40 in D and £24.00 in F. In E the charge was £4.50 of people's DLA with nothing more for those on Income Support, but up to a maximum of £225 for people with higher incomes or capital.

People getting ILF awards tended to buy assistance up to the level of those awards, not always spending their assessed contribution on care but very often doing so and sometimes also spending on additional hours from their own pockets. Both LA and ILF charges were resented when people were having to find extra money from their own resources either to pay for extra help when that was needed but not included in their regular package, or to pay for various expenses associated with having assistance.

Summary

Social services budget constraints have led to contractions in services and waiting lists for equipment; the prioritisation of assessment over ongoing support and review; and the imposition of ceilings on expenditure on individual community care packages. Consequently, some people are having to make do with less support than they need and some are getting inappropriate services.

Expenditure ceilings are set with reference to the cost of residential/nursing homecare, but the ILF 93 Fund threshold of £200 for social services contributions, its maximum of £300 for its own contribution and the £500 ceiling it imposes for the joint cost of packages for new applicants also have a significant impact on how these ceilings are set and how they operate. The national £500 limit disadvantages those living in high-cost areas. Ceilings are imposed less rigidly for people under 65 than for older people, but care managers now have much less discretion than previously to agree high-cost packages.

Sometimes there is an incentive to use in-house homecare or day centre provision because these either are not subject to critical budget ceilings or else make the ILF threshold easier to reach.

Local authorities have to consider spending more than £200 a week where a person is not eligible for the ILF, where such an application is not appropriate, or where the ILF is contributing its maximum but the overall cost is increasing to above £500. They have to consider covering the *full* cost of packages assessed at over £500 if there is not already an ILF contribution.

Social services responses to such situations are variable. There are cases where discretion to spend the necessary amount is agreed (especially, but not always, where the only residential care considered appropriate is even more expensive), and others where the person has to go into cheaper residential care. In many cases, packages are contained within £500 by means that lead to inadequate and unsatisfactory outcomes acceptable to disabled people only because the alternative is residential care.

6
Assistance with personal care

This chapter is concerned with the construction of support packages that help people with their personal care: that is, essential everyday tasks such as dressing, eating, washing, toileting, getting in and out of bed and moving around. Other aspects of social care and a further examination of issues related to choice and control are dealt with in Chapter 8. Here, we consider the benefits achieved by different arrangements and the compromises made in order to keep overall costs within applied financial limits.

Complexity of arrangements

People with high support needs often have complicated support packages, sometimes with a full mix of social services Homecare, independent sector agencies and private personal assistance. Day centre and regular respite in residential settings may be provided in addition and district nurses may visit. Although the latter are not included in social care costs, their available input is an important consideration when packages are constructed (see Chapter 7).

An example of a particularly complex care package was provided by **Len**, who had cerebral palsy and lived with his mother who was in poor health. Len attended a day centre five days a week (funded jointly by LA/HA), had social services Homecarers helping him get up and go to bed each day and 40 other day hours a week from an agency (funded by the ILF Extension Fund). Two other agencies each provided help for sessions of a few hours each week (also ILF funded). Social services currently provided a sleepover care assistant two nights a week from its small night

care service while his mother recovered from an operation, and up to seven nights a month were spent in respite care (with DSS funding to which there were preserved rights dating from before 1993). No overall limit was thus set on Len's care costs, which were shared between the LA, HA, DSS, ILF Extension Fund and Len himself. The arrangement was particularly complicated for the ILF, which had to adjust its payments to cover extra agency hours each time Len was unable to go to the day centre or for respite. This was happening frequently because he was prone to chest infections.

Most of the disabled people covered in our research were getting less than this wide range of inputs, but a combination of private and agency assistance, for example, was common and, in some areas, in-house services covered certain slots while agencies covered others. These mixtures of provision often meant that many different workers were coming into the disabled person's house every week.

In the same authority as Len, **Jenny** had help from social services, the NHS and the ILF 93 Fund and was grateful for the combination of services, which had enabled her to stay in the community when her husband died. She needed a significant amount of assistance for she was paraplegic and needed tube feeding. She also suffered from osteoporosis, diabetes and epilepsy. It had been suggested that she go into a nursing home once her husband went into hospital, but she knew that this would be an irrevocable decision and preferred to remain in her own home for a while until she had coped with her bereavement and was ready to make decisions about her future. However, she had found the pattern of her support package frustrating:

> "It's rather like I'm institutionalised in my own home. That's how I feel. It's sort of times for this, times for that, certain times to get up, certain times to go to bed, whether you want to or not. I can't have any say about the times the nurses come.... What I miss is quality time. There's get-ups, there's overnights and that's it. And it's very wearing when you have so many people coming through the door in 24 hours, a constant flow of people. They're asking you things and you're having to repeat the same things over and over. Sometimes I just feel like telling them to go away."

The obvious questions raised by this are: why are some support packages so complicated and are they necessarily so? And why are particular types of provision chosen?

In some cases, such as that of Len, one answer is that the package has evolved over a number of years as circumstances have changed. Arrangements that seem to work well, or are familiar, or simply are available, are added to rather than replaced and the result is a patchwork of provision which may or may not be cost-effective. However, another answer is that particular types of provision are associated with particular sources of funding and policies of the funders, for example, in-house services are insisted upon by a LA, ILF money cannot be used for in-house services, the NHS will pay only for its own district nurses, etc. The outcome for Jenny is somewhat less than ideal.

Live-in support

One way of avoiding some of the problems described above is to have a live-in assistant whose availability offers the flexibility that many people with high support needs find difficult to get with a patchwork of different service providers. Live-in support can also be cheaper, a

number of agencies being able to offer it within £500 (in some areas at least). It depends on the nature and frequency of the assistance that is needed and in particular upon the need for help during the night. A package for less than £500 might be possible, for example, if one assistant can cope for several days at a time and rotate with one or two others, or if one person works for several weeks or months with appropriate periods of relief covered by other workers.

The cheapest provision that commercial agencies can offer is an introductory service, where workers are self-employed and only an introductory fee for each one recruited is charged, rather than ongoing agency administration costs plus VAT. Two might, for example, be recruited to work alternate weeks. This arrangement may be appropriate where the physical demands on the worker are not very great and where there is infrequent need for active assistance during the night. In some areas, however, it is difficult to recruit live-in assistance. Reasons vary, but bad housing conditions and rough areas are important deterrents.

We came across two types of agency that employed young people as low-cost, short-term, live-in assistants. One of our authorities had been paying for Community Service Volunteers (CSVs), but was currently stopping these arrangements because of the extra monitoring and support that was being required of its social workers. Ten people in this authority had been using CSVs and all but one had now finished. The second type of agency recruited travellers from overseas who were willing to work for several months at a time and often had relevant experience. In the London borough and the rural authority in our study, this was the only way that 24-hour cover could be afforded for less than £500 a week.

In Authority E, a not-for-profit agency supplying live-in workers had been set up within the previous year to recruit assistants for disabled people who were getting indirect payments. A 10-hour day and sleepover was required of each worker and negotiations with relatives and friends were carried out to help cover relief gaps. This enabled the agency to keep the overall cost just within £500. The cost broke down into £415 for the worker, £50 for National Insurance (NI) and £60 for the agency's administration, the user paying the balance from their DLA. The arrangements had been largely successful, but there was some concern about what would happen to people as their condition deteriorated and more help was needed (for example, two people for lifting).

The limitations with this sort of provision lie in the youth and lack of continuity of the assistants. The arrangement may work well for some younger clients wanting assistants of around the same age, but not for people wanting more maturity and continuity.

Brian had used CSVs for 20 years, many from overseas who were able to take advantage of the local language school while he was at work. He had taken on about 100 different assistants over that period. Unlike another CSV-user in the same area who had 11 workers during the 18 months after leaving residential care, seven of whom were unsatisfactory, Brian's experience had been largely positive.

> "I would say I can think of only three where it hasn't really worked. However, as the years go by, the gap between myself and my helpers is getting bigger in terms of basically just what makes you tick. I think if you are going to live in the same house as somebody in a fairly intimate environment, you want to be able to interrelate even if they're not necessary your friends or colleagues. And the interests of the average 20-year-old are not the interests of your average 40-year-old. So I've come to the conclusion that it's time to change."

In principle, Brian's particular circumstances should mean that he will be able to arrange a rota of live-in carers through an agency for less than £400 a week. His initial contacts with a number of agencies had confirmed this but also revealed that the agencies varied greatly in the extent to which he would be allowed to be involved in the selection process. Recruitment was proving difficult, however, possibly because of his requirement that his assistants should be drivers.

Live-in arrangements are usually considered only where the disabled person lives alone. It is otherwise likely to be an unacceptably intrusive arrangement for a parent or partner. Even then, for such an arrangement to be successful, there has to be suitable accommodation, usually a separate bedroom, and this is not always available. Although the problem is now better understood, it continues to be difficult for a disabled person to find suitable two-bedroomed accommodation and people leaving the parental home or coming out of residential care often fail to anticipate a future need for live-in assistance.

Independent living and privacy

There are disadvantages as well as advantages from the perspective of someone with high support needs in having live-in assistance. The problem stems from the lack of privacy. A number of our interviewees expressed the concern that they felt little enough control in their lives already and that having someone with them in their house all the time was too much of an intrusion. Where 24-hour attention was necessary because of physical risk, there might be little choice, but otherwise time alone was important. Some people found themselves negotiating *down* their assessed hours because of this.

> "Just recently I had a reassessment of my care package and the social worker was quite worried that I might be putting myself at risk by getting into bed at the end of the day on my own, because I do have osteoporosis as well as multiple sclerosis.

But I like my independence and the thought of having someone watching the same television programmes that you are watching, just hovering around for the time you need to go to the toilet, or the time you want to go to bed.... She wanted to increase my hours into the evening, but it was important for me to keep a little bit of my own real independence, the fact that I'm on my own and that's what I want." (Pat)

Others talked of the need for "having the house to myself and some breathing space"; "not being molly coddled or fussed over"; "having your own life". **Pauline** said that she really needed more assistance, "but on the other hand, it's silly to say, but it's a bit of an imposition when you've got folks coming in four times a day. You feel the house isn't your own any more". **Mary** liked to maintain gaps between the assistants so that she did not feel totally "taken over".

Sue was aware that she could have a live-in assistant for the same money she was paying for her current package, but decided to have a catheter so that she could do without having people around her all the time and could be alone at night. There was no medical need for catheterisation, but she was unable to get to the toilet without help.

Mike's doctor had told him that he needed live-in care, but he was concerned about the narrow range of people willing to do that sort of work. At least with the friends who were currently employed as personal assistants, he had some choice among people he knew and liked.

There was, however, the danger that if a person once refused an offer of extra hours, it might prove difficult to get them when they *were* wanted:

"We cut it down because I don't want people around me all day. But, because we once said no, when you do need it they say you can't have it unless you pay extortionate prices." (William)

Sometimes, a satisfactory arrangement for those wanting privacy was to have an assistant living nearby with a pager, on call during set hours rather than constantly present.

Night-time assistance

It was difficult for people to get night-time care. A number of those we interviewed felt that they did need someone with them at night, but were having to accept a compromise.

William's night care was funded by the ILF 93 Fund but, because he had to be turned every two hours, this was waking night care and expensive. He was therefore having only six hours a night in order to afford it within the Fund's maximum £300 a week, but that meant staying up until midnight, which was sometimes difficult.

Robert, in the same authority, also needed frequent help during the night, but having an Extension Fund award of £455 on top of his social services assistance meant that he did not have to restrict his number of hours. **Martha**, also with an Extension Fund award of £400, was able to afford seven nights of cover.

Hilary found that, because her condition varied a great deal, she needed to use her ILF award and social services direct payments flexibly to make sure that she could cover her need for the occasional extra night. She would have to compensate by having fewer day hours. There was some extra contingency money attached to her direct payments but that was not supposed to be used for night care, so she did not have the total flexibility she would have liked.

A social services nightwatch service was provided two nights a week for **Len** to give his mother some undisturbed sleep. She would normally be up four times a night. The service had been provided for the previous six years and was highly valued but it had been reduced recently from three to two nights.

Mike's assessed care package was just under £500 a week and part of the ILF 93 Fund award was supposed to pay for four nights, but Mike had not been able to afford four nights and could cover them only by reducing day-time hours. His assessment had originally identified a need for seven nights but had subsequently been reduced in order to stay within the £500 limit.

Support from in-house Homecare

In four of the six authorities, there was a general policy of 'in-house first' and use of the independent sector had to be justified when getting a care package authorised. As mentioned in Chapter 5, these policies were more rigidly imposed in some areas than others, even within the same authority. Elsewhere, it was acknowledged that the in-house service was primarily a service for older people and that younger disabled people were less likely to have to use it. The 'hidden cost' of an in-house service could, however, be an incentive when putting together a high support package (see Chapter 5). Also, some social workers expressed regret that, with a much reduced in-house service, they had lost the opportunity they once had to use it as a reliable fall-back in an emergency.

In Authority F, the in-house Homecare service had moved away from providing domestic cleaning towards the provision of high levels of personal care. Social workers considered its staff to be of high quality and particularly good for complex needs and terminal care. The problem concerned flexibility of time. Technically the service could be provided only between 7am and 10pm and not on bank holidays, unless the package normally contained weekend cover. Also, in-house provision was based upon the completion of tasks, whereas outside agencies were commissioned for full hours. Users could get more out of agencies than out of Homecare, where tasks were often rushed. One Homecarer might be responsible for 10 get-ups. This authority, like some others, was struggling to

make its in-house service more flexible both to complement and to compete with the independent sector.

In-house Homecare was often described as a 'doing' rather than an 'enabling' service, revealing its links to the original home help services, but there were variations. In Authority B, for example, a Homecarer would not be able to take the user out, whereas in Authority F this was acceptable. These differences impacted on disabled people's aspirations to independent living.

> *"I wanted help to do the shopping, but Homecare workers won't come with you to do the shopping. They will do the shopping for you, which seems absolutely stupid because you can't have any involvement in what's being bought for you. People think I'm nuts but I like going shopping because I can feel the vegetables and the fruit. It's about choice again. You don't always know in advance what you want do you."* **(Pat)**

> *"They want to get somebody to get Jimmy into bed at 9 o'clock. My argument is his life is over if he's got to go to bed at 9 o'clock. He goes to bed at 11 purely for me because by 11 o'clock I've had enough. It would be a really good thing if I could get someone to come at 11 or a little bit later to put Jim to bed, but they haven't got carers that will come."* **(Jim's mother)**

Although there was a general consensus about the inflexibility of rules governing in-house services, only a minority of our interviewees were now using these services. Most used independent sector agencies or employed personal assistants with direct or indirect payments.

Support from independent sector agencies

Praise of and complaints about independent sector agencies varied both within and between different authorities. On the positive side they could provide flexible times, carefully selected staff, involvement of the user, consistency, good management and willingness to train for tasks such as help with physiotherapy. On the negative side there were complaints about badly trained staff, lack of continuity, high turnover, unreliability, etc.

In rural Authority A, agencies found it difficult to recruit staff because the low wages they offered meant that many people were better off on benefit. The rates agencies had to charge were nonetheless high because of travel costs. One third of the agency costs for one of our interviewees was travel costs. There were problems in rural areas of finding assistants with relevant skills who did not have to travel from some distance. Also reasons to do with privacy and confidentiality meant that people who lived in the same small village were often not acceptable. It was therefore difficult to find agencies able to provide for people with high support needs for under £500. The availability of emergency cover was also an issue because of the distances involved.

In Authority D, there had been a large number of contracts with small agencies, but the social services list had recently been reduced, many agencies choosing not to invest the amount necessary to meet requirements without any guarantee of getting work (just as the new list came out, the budget was frozen and there was no new work anyway). Within social services it was suggested that a number of smaller, cheaper, good-quality agencies had dropped off the list for this reason, an observation supported by discussions with people in the private sector who claimed that the costs of administering the monitoring, tendering and accreditation data required by the authority were prohibitive for small agencies, which faced none of this with their private clients. There was also concern about the inflexibility of contracts. It was suggested that when clients wanted small changes to the arrangements initially agreed with their care

managers, this often involved protracted renegotiations.

In Authority B, social services staff were supposed to look for the cheapest agency first and all agency provision was spot-purchased. In Authority E, there were 10 agencies on the approved list, three of which had service-level agreements. The others were used for spot contracts. In Authority F, there was a mixture of block and spot contracts and a recent move away from an 'in-house first' policy; 15 agencies were on the approved list. In Authority C, there had until recently been a long list of independent providers, but many were now going out of business or failing to meet social services requirements. There was one list of cheaper accredited agencies and another of more expensive ones. Care managers were supposed to try two from the cheaper list before using a more expensive agency. Only two independent sector agencies had block contracts. Again, staff were instructed to try Homecare first and in this authority had to put requests even for this service before a panel, but Homecare tended to be fully committed and unable to take on big packages.

Although some among our disabled interviewees had criticisms of the private agencies they had experienced (and in one authority in particular, criticisms heavily outweighed praise), others were fully satisfied with their arrangements. Some, such as **Ahmed**, felt that disabled people were now more able to challenge practices knowing that agencies were in competition with each other and as a result had become more responsive to disabled people's requirements:

> *"Their attitudes towards providing care workers seem to be different. I don't know whether it's across the board, whether they're actually using that new philosophy to help other disabled people, but when it comes to me, they're quite open minded and flexible. But it also seems that the more information disabled people have and the*

more they can disseminate it, the more they can challenge people ... so the care managers or the owners of care agencies sometimes feel quite defensive, which actually I think is quite a good idea because they know that the person who wants the care knows what they're talking about."

The description of independent sector agency use in this section was based on snapshots during 1998. In most of these authorities the picture was one of flux, with both confusion and apprehension about changes in policies which might offer higher quality and more flexible services, but might also restrict the scope of social workers who had to arrange high support packages. The effects of pressure from some SSDs to negotiate low rates and restrict their lists of accredited providers were evident.

Caroline had been forced to change to a cheaper agency but feared that she would soon be losing her care workers who could be earning higher wages with the first agency, now off the approved list because of its cost.

"Before I joined [name of agency], I was with another one which paid their helpers more and seemed to get a slightly higher quality of carers. But they put their prices up and social services wouldn't increase their money, so I had to swap agencies. What do people like me do?"

Support from directly recruited personal assistants

ILF clients have been able to recruit and employ their own personal assistants since the original Fund started operating in 1988. As detailed in Chapter 3, some of our interviewees were now employing personal assistants with money from the 93 Fund or the Extension Fund, others with indirect or direct LA payments and some with both ILF and LA funding. These arrangements offered the choice and control that many disabled people wanted. Although allocated a budget based on a certain number of hours of assistance at a

certain price, they were usually able to use that budget flexibly to change details of times and rates to suit themselves and to adjust these from week to week through direct negotiations with the assistants they employed.

No interviewees who were getting direct or indirect payments wanted to return to social services provision. Like **Dora**, they found that not only were they now getting more assistance for the money available, but the quality of that assistance suited them much better:

"I suffered tremendously when I was under social services because it wasn't a consistent sort of arrangement. You had different people coming in and out, they paid them and they have these agencies. You didn't get involved with the carers and this was very, very bad. You need someone who can understand your cultural needs and all this sort of thing. So this corrected itself when I got the care brokerage.... Before I went onto care brokerage, the money I got didn't cover the hours I'm entitled to. Compared with what I had before I'm a lot more satisfied."

Dora was from an ethnic minority group and found a particular advantage in the flexibility of being able to recruit her own assistants. In another of our six authorities, where there was a high proportion of ethnic minority residents, there was a concern that only a very small number had as yet come onto the indirect payments scheme.

In Authority E, where there had been 35 to 40 indirect payments recipients, many of whom would be converting to direct payments during 1998, social services staff did not assume that these packages would be cheaper than service provision. In theory, at least, if a slightly higher cost would significantly enhance a person's quality of life, then this would be acceptable. In practice, because eligibility for indirect payments was restricted to people who qualified for help from the ILF, then the £500 limit had to apply (at least when the package was first set up).

Authority A was also developing a direct payments scheme based upon the experience of making a small number of indirect payments for some years. As in Authority E, social services funded a support scheme in the voluntary sector which currently worked with 13 people. A senior manager within the department expressed the view that recipients of the original direct payments were people who were particularly capable of organising their own assistance and determined to do so and it was unlikely that there were many others who would be willing to take on the responsibility. Payments were calculated on the assumption that recipients would not be using them to pay agencies, and extra money for agency VAT was disallowed. Within the voluntary sector organisation, it was felt that many more people would want to move from service provision to direct payments if the support scheme could act as employer for them for an interim period as they moved more gradually towards full independent living. The problem with this option for people with high-level needs would be that the scheme might itself become VAT liable and the cost of some packages be taken above allowable limits.

There was considerable variation, both across and within the different SSDs, when it came to care managers' enthusiasm for direct payments. In Authority B, where 50 direct payments were expected to be established by April 1998, one care manager said that *all* the disabled people she worked with had been transferred onto direct payments ("It's difficult to kick in but it works"). However, she added that there was considerable difficulty getting the idea promoted in some other areas of the authority, where there remained a strong insistence upon using in-house services wherever possible.

In newly unitary Authority F, indirect payments, of which there were now 22, had been inherited from the previous administration and there was a plan to operate a direct payments scheme from 1999, but, again, there was resistance from many care managers ("There's a potential for irregularities and staff don't want to get bogged down").

In Authority C, three different voluntary sector organisations offered brokerage for a small number of people getting indirect payments from social services (most of these arrangements were initiated in the 1980s at levels now unavailable for new packages because of budget constraints). A pilot direct payments project had been agreed. In Authority D, a pilot indirect payments project had been running for a year but with limited success because of resistance from social workers, lack of adequate structural support and minimal promotion to encourage service users to explore the option.

Clearly, direct payments were not always presented in ways that would encourage rather than discourage participants. Opinion within social services divided between those who thought that few disabled people (and even fewer over 65) would want direct payments, and those who thought that take-up depended entirely upon how well the idea was promoted. Low predictions of numbers leading to low limits on direct payments budgets presented a 'catch-22'.

"I said to the lady at the town hall 'Why don't you have an awareness week?' And they said 'It would be dreadful to make them aware and then we can't give it to them'." (Jane)

Our interviews in all six authorities revealed that, although people who received ILF awards and/or direct or indirect payments from social services were able to avoid agency commission and VAT by employing their own personal assistants, some with high needs still struggled to keep costs within the amount they had been allocated, and in particular within the crucial limit of £500 (for various of the reasons covered in Chapter 4 and later in Chapter 8).

Social services and disabled people themselves were using a variety of means to try to constrain overall costs. Apart from the reductions in day hours or numbers of nights mentioned before, they variously left gaps between assistants wherever possible, did not pay new assistants when they were learning alongside more experienced ones, did not pay cost of living increases, had the administration charges of support schemes waived in order to keep under the £500, and generally cut corners on their activities.

Employing friends or relations as personal assistants sometimes made it easier to tailor a high support package to fit under the £500 ceiling because their goodwill could be tapped. **Margaret**, for example, had been in hospital for three years since a road traffic accident. Returning home to an adapted house, she was assessed as needing 60.5 day hours and seven nights of assistance. The original plan was to pay a friend and her son £5 an hour and £32 per night (the rates suggested by the ILF), with allowances for bank holidays and other holidays, but this had failed to take into account employer NI. The rate paid for night care was therefore reduced to £25 and a final overall cost of £564.85 agreed (Margaret paying the balance of £64.85, which was just a few pence more than the personal contribution required by the ILF's normal financial assessment).

New Working Time Regulations and the National Minimum Wage

One agency employed by an interviewee calculated that the new Working Time Regulations (WTR), which came into force in October 1998, would add 6.12% to its wage costs.

This was because it would then start paying for three weeks' holiday a year to staff who had previously been employed on a casual basis. From October 1999, the requirement of four weeks' annual holiday would increase that percentage to 8.33. The United Kingdom Home Care Association (UKHCA) has suggested that the WTR effects are likely to vary significantly by region and the Local Government Association has recommended that renegotiations of contracts be conducted on a local basis (Laing & Buisson, 1998b). Similarly, the National Minimum Wage (NMW) is likely to have a different impact by region and it is difficult to predict the extent to which domiciliary care costs will be affected. There will also be an impact on residential and nursing home fees and thus on some of the comparisons made between costs of placements and community care costs.

The possible implications of these two new measures were only beginning to be appreciated during the period of the research, but some concern was expressed that the arrangements of live-in care assistants might be affected by the new regulations on numbers of hours worked per average week. Few disabled people expressed much knowledge of the new regulations but a number of them were aware that currently they were not able to treat their employees in the way they felt they should be able to:

> "I can't afford to pay them holiday pay out of that money, so if somebody has a holiday, they fill in for each other and that kind of tops up their normal hours. I would like to be able to pay them holiday pay but funds don't allow." **(Julie)**

When people received LA direct payments there was sometimes an allowance for holiday pay built into the package, but longer-established ILF awards (Extension or 93 Fund) did not contain that provision. Most people were unaware that, provided they were not already getting the maximum award, they could now ask the ILF for an increase to cover any extra costs raised by the WTR or NMW.

It is perhaps worth bearing in mind that 24-hour care calculated at a NMW of £3.60 an hour would cost £604.80 a week.

Lifting, moving and handling

The introduction of European Union regulations about lifting and handling has had a significant impact on people with high support needs. It has created major problems for social workers trying to keep the costs of packages within certain limits and frustrations for disabled people who have had their activity curtailed.

In the past in Authority B, social services care managers turned to independent sector agencies when domiciliary care involved lifting, because the in-house service applied a 'no-lift' policy. Recently, however, accredited agencies had become subject to the same rules and social services had instructed its staff that, where two people were needed for lifting, they should request help from the community nursing service. Getting this sort of help from district nurses was not easy (see Chapter 7). The 'no-lift' rule also contributed to the constraints upon a night-time service offered by the department. This sitting service could be provided only where an informal carer was present in the house, so that there was a second person available to help with lifting and handling if necessary. It could never be provided for a disabled person living alone.

Laura used to be able to use a standing frame when she lived with her parents because her father would help one of her assistants to get her onto it. Now, however, in her own home, she had only one assistant at a time:

"Now, there's all this red tape. It's a big no-no. Because I have only one Homecarer in the morning, she's not able to lift me into the standing frame. So the standing frame is a big no-

no and I don't stand so well and I'm probably going to get osteoporosis of the bones.... When I was in [name of respite residence] I asked and they were trying to sort me out an electrical standing frame. They tried it out on me. It works but it's an expensive contraption and funding let the whole thing down."

An example was given by a care manager who had begun to wonder whether one young disabled person had not had a more enriching life in the residential home she had left than in the community since 'no-lift' policies had been implemented. This young woman was 21 years old and weighed only 6 stone. Overlaps of her live-in assistants could be arranged for lifting times, but there could be no lifting without a hoist. This meant that she could not go out if it meant being away from the hoist for more than two hours. She could not use pads because of pressure sores but would not have wanted to anyway.

The new lifting regulations, exacerbated by cuts in staff, also meant that people who needed more attention were less likely to be offered places at day centres in Authority A (see Chapter 8 for other consequences of restricted day centre opportunities).

Here and elsewhere it was suggested, by both care managers and disabled interviewees alike, that restrictions on lifting were forcing some people to lose their ability to walk and to become fully dependent upon wheelchairs much earlier than would otherwise have been the case.

"I could stand and transfer with a bit of help, from the bed to the wheelchair and from the wheelchair to the loo. The carers who came were managing alright, you know. They didn't actually have to lift me up but they had to help me get onto my feet. But the care manager arrived one afternoon and she said she wasn't prepared to put any carers in because of the sort of personal

handling arrangements. She wanted a hoist installed and refused to send in carers unless there was a hoist installed. And that upset me because there was no consultation with me. She didn't ask me what my opinion was. And I knew that if I got a hoist in the house, it would mean the end of my standing, if you like. And I saw that as a way of making my disability worse sooner than it needed to have been. I could see that at some stage in the future I would have needed a hoist, but while I was still able to do some sort of movement and standing with help, I felt I was being discriminated against for the benefit of the agency." ***(Pauline)***

One social worker in Authority F had noticed a jump in the cost of some packages as a direct result of moving and handling regulations. He himself had only just discovered that, even if a disabled person had a ceiling track hoist, two assistants were supposed to be provided for lifting. He was about to examine the care packages of six service users where, if this was necessary, the cost of the package would increase above the department's ceiling.

In Authority E, issues around lifting and handling for people in receipt of indirect and direct payments were unresolved and there was some concern about the authority's liability where users refused to use hoists or have a second assistant for lifting. Responsibility for risk assessment had been passed to users. It was recognised at the same time that the ILF did not demand assurances on employee health and safety at any time after their initial assessment of need, so there was the potential for confusion for jointly funded packages if social services insisted upon restrictions. It was generally the case that people getting indirect or direct payments had more flexibility and autonomy in the arrangements they agreed with their employees, but there was some social services concern about this.

Summary

Some community care packages are complex patchworks of different provision which may have evolved over a number of years as circumstances have changed, or else are the consequence of restrictive policies and practices of funding agencies. In either case, questions have to be asked about whether the package is best value for the disabled person. Far from enhancing independence, some arrangements of services can exclude people from participating in normal everyday life.

Live-in support can be cheaper and may be ideal if the person wants younger assistants. But it is not always feasible because of housing constraints or recruitment problems. It may not be desirable either, privacy being a quality that people with high support needs often value highly but find difficult to secure.

Night-time cover is an area where people make major compromises in order to stay within available budgets. This is a particular problem when waking nights are involved. Some people with Extension Fund awards, where higher ceilings apply, can more easily afford night care.

The 'in-house first' policy operated in some authorities tends to be applied less rigidly to under-65s, but where it is applied the inflexibility of the service is significant. Disabled people's experience of independent sector agencies is very varied and in some authorities much better than others. There is sometimes concern about the development of restricted lists of accredited agencies and its effect on the scope of social workers to arrange high support packages, also on the disabled people forced to change to cheaper agencies.

Those with ILF awards or social services direct payments value the choice and control these bring, including their ability to choose ways of 'cutting corners' in order to keep under the £500 ceiling.

Although direct payments schemes are being developed, this is against the resistance of some social services staff and clearly direct payments are not always presented in ways which encourage rather than discourage participants. Low predictions of numbers leading to low direct payments budgets and cautious promotion present a 'catch-22' situation.

The introduction of lifting restrictions has increased the cost of community care for people with high support needs and created frustrations for those whose activities have been curtailed. The National Minimum Wage and Working Time Regulations are developments also likely to raise costs. All these changes, although having the potential for raising standards, make it increasingly difficult to contain costs within current LA and ILF ceilings.

7

Assistance with healthcare

The social/healthcare divide

Some of the most expensive community care packages are considered viable only because there is a key health service input, either of NHS funded and arranged community nursing, day centre provision and respite, or through some joint funding whereby the social/healthcare divide is bridged. Continuing (long-term) care criteria, agreed locally between LAs and HAs, form the basis upon which the latter can happen, but the interpretation of existing criteria is constantly debated. Our research revealed wide variations in policy and practice in this area impinging strongly upon the opportunities of people with physical impairments and high support needs. We came across many examples of social services care managers struggling to put together acceptable arguments for health service support to make these high support packages financially viable. It seemed to be in this area, rather than in the area of learning disabilities or mental health, that the social/healthcare divide operated at its worst in terms of outcomes for users.

Arguments such as: "Where any individual community care package costs more than £500 a week, there should be some health authority involvement" (SSD senior manager) met with the response: "The criteria are about recognising needs, not simply looking for funding for a high cost package" (HA service development manager). The problem was that 'needs' were related to available services rather than to outcomes for the user.

At a strategic level, Authority E, where the above comments were made, had successfully insisted that health service funding should not be restricted to care by qualified nurses, allowing for the possibility of other care workers being trained to perform tasks that were arguably healthcare responsibilities (for example, night-time turning or gastrostomy feeding). However, every case had to be argued separately to the continuing care panel and the problem for people under 65 was that there was no multidisciplinary team or assessment system able to coordinate such a request. Needs were not assessed prior to crises developing, at which point requests for health funding were rejected on the grounds that it was purely a 'single party' social services assessment with evidence for healthcare needs not adequately demonstrated. Efforts to clarify and improve this situation were in progress but by the end of 1998 there was still only one example of NHS funding of any provision that was not both arranged and managed within the NHS itself (and this for nursing agency provision). Here and elsewhere, it was felt that the holistic approach to care management essential for someone with both health and social care needs was lacking and much better systems of joint working were required. In one area, we were told of "games being played" to get health service funding by ploys such as writing 'terminal' on application forms, but this tended to rebound because the case would then be considered short-term and there would be inadequate planning for the future.

In Authority D, a policy document had been jointly published four years previously by the LA and four local HAs to define in a detailed and practical way the boundary between social care and nursing care. However, this was now felt to be inadequate, there being no consistency in how certain needs such as two-person lifting and tube feeding were addressed. The more recent continuing care criteria, written by the HA, had been noted rather than formally agreed by the LA. In the words of a senior social services manager, "We are striving towards a mutual understanding, but we have the social bath controversy at regular intervals!"

In Authority A, there was no NHS continuing care funding for older or physically disabled people in the community ("The continuing care criteria were written by the health authority and are so tight that hardly anyone who isn't in a nursing home or dying can get help" - senior social services manager). There was also a low level of district nurse services and, as a consequence, some of the tasks being taken on by social services funded agencies were nursing tasks. This had sometimes been concealed, for example, when an agency provided a nurse for the cost of an auxiliary. In social services it was felt that there was little health service commitment to the maintenance of a person's life-style. The difference in approach was demonstrated when a local resettlement programme for people moving back into the community after a spinal injury had produced resettlement proposals that were greatly at variance with community nursing assessments for the same individuals.

When we interviewed in Authority F, there was just one case of continuing care funding being put towards a community package. This was seen by the care manager as "uncharted territory". In general, a justification for distinctive health (as opposed to social) care was required and any assumption by social services staff that continuing care funding should be sought where the cost of package exceeded £500 was disputed. There had been a revision of the health and social care protocol in 1997 but social workers still experienced wide variations in interpretation by district nurses from one health centre to another,

some being willing to be much more flexible than others.

There were good reasons for social workers to try to get an NHS contribution towards a high support package. With ceilings on both social services expenditure and joint funding with the ILF, it could mean the difference between someone staying in the community and going into a nursing home. But, apart from narrow interpretations of continuing care criteria and the roles of different care workers, several other barriers were in the way of constructive and creative community support across the divide. Examples were:

- Problems were faced in setting up and administering joint LA and HA funding of packages when one contribution was subject to charges to the user and the other not.

- Direct payments presented a conflict of interests because NHS money could not be used to pay for assistants employed by the disabled person themselves.

- A related issue concerned ILF applications. Getting NHS funding or provision for part of a package could crucially bring the balance that had to be funded by social services to below £500 and an ILF award might then allow the social services contribution to be as low as £200. Health authority funding might thus enable someone to access the ILF, with all the choice and control this offered, but the person would have to accept that part of their package could not be arranged through direct or indirect payments but would have to be arranged through less flexible health services, that is, through an agency or community nursing.

Developments in two of our six authorities had cut through some of these barriers.

In **Authority B**, the Healthcare Development Manager noted that training non-qualified care workers to mobilise and feed people well could be very cost-effective, but it was essential to have continuity, which was always difficult with agency staff. In her opinion, being able to fund dedicated care staff through direct payments could help overcome this problem and it was acknowledged that already the direct payments scheme run by social services was contributing to the physio-maintenance of individuals in a way that the community nursing mainstream services could not.

In the early stages of our research there was already one case in this authority where continuing care money was being used to support someone in the community through a package fully paid for through direct payments. In this case, social services were invoicing the HA on a monthly basis and there was no problem about charges because direct payments recipients were exempt.

Later, other jointly funded direct payments packages were being set up on the same basis and a policy had developed whereby a community care package could attract NHS funding on the basis of needs for turning, lifting by more than one person and psycho-social needs. A trade-off was increasingly being acknowledged for the expanding number of people getting direct payments. Where costs were above £500, the HA was coming in with funding and where costs were below £500, personal assistants recruited by disabled people and funded by social services were being trained for tasks that might otherwise have been expected of the health service, for example, the tasks mentioned above plus things such as catheter care and physiotherapy.

Ironically, having achieved the key element of health funding, one problem that now existed with these arrangements was that the HA

contribution was the only one (unlike the LA and ILF contributions) where an inflationary element was built in whereas both the social services and ILF contributions were limited by ceilings.

In **Authority C**, there was a good example of effective joint working by social services and the health authority in the Community Multiple Sclerosis (MS) Team. The collaboration between the two authorities in this health trust-funded team (supported by the MS Society) meant that access to the full range of social and medical services could be shared. Occupational therapy, physiotherapy, counselling, social work, psychology and medical services were all offered within the team, with referral to other services also possible. This was all without the need for an individual's GP to be involved. There were thus better opportunities for monitoring changes in needs once care packages were set up and more coordination, flexibility, speed and innovation (for example, with problems associated with fatigue) could be provided.

In practice, the volume of referrals of people with MS and the complexity of their needs were outstripping the team social worker's ability to take on referrals, and these were having to be prioritised within social services first. Our interviews with disabled people in the area confirmed satisfaction with the high level of support provided for those people with MS fortunate enough to be referred to the team compared with the level of support available to some other disabled people in the same authority (compare **Jacqueline** with **Ian** below).

The existence of the MS Team, despite its inability to meet demand, compensated to some extent for certain problems likely to be faced by people with MS, for example, the fact that there was often a working husband or wife so the ILF means-test would deter people from wanting to apply to the Fund, or the variability of their condition, which sometimes made it difficult to get the higher rate of the DLA care component, a necessary eligibility criteria for ILF help.

Despite the success of the MS Team, it had not become any easier for other physically disabled people with high support needs in Authority C to get HA funding. It was suggested, for example, that there was a large number of people with brain injuries in residential care locally who could have lived in the community given an equivalent level of support.

Physiotherapy

The service provided by the MS Team in Authority C highlighted the difficulty elsewhere of getting the level of physiotherapy that disabled people felt they needed, particularly people with MS. Sometimes, suggested one specialist care manager, this was because social workers failed to recognise the sort of help disabled people required. The example he gave was of a man who would be able to go out in the car with his personal assistant if only he could be given more practice in transferring. At other times it was simply that the community physiotherapy service operated at too low a level and was difficult to access.

The opinion of many of the disabled people we interviewed was that regular physiotherapy was a high priority for them and they wanted more than they were able to get. Examples have already been given in Chapter 6 of people unable to use their standing frames to get exercise because of lifting regulations. Others had had six weeks of treatment with the idea that they would continue the exercises, but they could not manage these by themselves.

In some cases there had been arrangements whereby care workers were trained to assist with the exercises, but the effectiveness of such an arrangement clearly depended upon a low turnover of workers.

"The local community physio was prepared to come in and show the morning carers what exercises to do. She was happy they were being done properly and I'm obviously happy that I'm getting them done regularly. But if someone strange was to come in they wouldn't know where to start." (Pauline)

Part of the negotiation for HA contribution towards Dan's direct payment care package concerned his need for regular physiotherapy. This had eventually been agreed and included a component for care workers trained by the community physiotherapist to provide this.

Case studies of people caught in the social/healthcare divide

Elisabeth

Elisabeth had joint SSD/ILF/HA funding for a 24-hour package costing roughly £1,000 a week, which was provided through a single nursing agency by three nurses and two care assistants. The qualified staff worked during the day-time and the unqualified staff at night. The only strict nursing procedure was the changing of a tracheostomy tube, which would normally happen at set times but was sometimes needed at other times if a problem arose. Our interview with Elisabeth and her sister, who was one of the nurses employed by the agency, revealed concern about the nights, when only untrained assistants were there.

"There should not be a time when Elisabeth is alone with a carer who cannot change her tracheostomy.... I'm telling the agency, but they've expressed to me their concern that the package is going over budget and they have to keep within budget. I would assume that if they're already over budget with three nurses and two carers, then to have five nurses would put them well over budget. So I think it's down to money."

It was also important that assistants were familiar with Elisabeth because her speech was difficult to understand, but getting familiar back-up staff through the agency when an assistant was off sick was always a problem. Elisabeth had heard of direct payments and thought that if she could recruit directly she would be able to afford five qualified nurses for the same total amount of money. But the various rules governing the three funding bodies would have made this impossible. Neither social services nor the ILF were supposed to fund nursing and the HA could not offer direct payments.

Christine

In Authority A there were inadequate community services for people with high support needs because of brain injuries or damage as a result of strokes, and care packages tended to break down. Christine's challenging behaviour meant that two care workers had to be present when her husband was not there. Support could not be provided through the learning disabilities team because her condition was acquired rather than congenital. It had proved impossible to arrange a day centre placement because the one-to-one attention Christine needed could not be provided, nor could a suitable residential home be found willing to have her for short respite stays to give her husband a break. The HA had agreed to pay for two nights a week for a temporary three-month period, but did not accept responsibility for ongoing funding which could have ensured a better-quality provision. The main problem from Christine and her husband's perspective was the number and turnover of different care workers and their lack of training:

"You get so many different carers, that's the trouble. I would say 8, 10, 12 a week and different each week. Once she gets used to one, they get moved on and we get another one. Half of them haven't got a clue when they get here, until she starts swearing at them and things like that and then they're taken aback.... They're not trained to

deal with anybody who has challenging behaviour and aren't told they're going to be dealing with someone with challenging behaviour. It can be very difficult."

Wendy

In Authority A, a 38-year-old woman with a brain tumour was in a nursing home because social services had imposed a strict limit on community care funding and was unwilling to pay more than £517, although she required only a few extra hours. The HA would not contribute any continuing care funding to community packages but was paying £310 towards the cost of the nursing home (social services paying the balance of £359) (source: SSD care manager).

Beth

Beth went into a nursing home from hospital respite eight years ago and stayed against her wishes because community care at home would cost more than £500. She was paying her DLA mobility component towards the £410 that the nursing home cost, the rest being covered by DSS preserved rights. Social services had argued that her needs were health-related but the HA would not agree to help fund a community care package. Beth had been fighting for the right to return to her fully adapted house, which had been empty for eight years. She felt that she had been pushed out of hospital into the nursing home too suddenly in the first place and then a series of obstacles put in her way to prevent her leaving.

"It's as if they're trying to frighten you out of wanting to go home because there's so much that could go wrong. But when I think of the things that have gone wrong since I've been in the home...."

A worker in a local voluntary organisation who knew Beth commented:

"The LA complaints system was used, but of course could not deal with the main issue which is

a disagreement with the decision not to award her a community care package. Unless the Gloucestershire judgment is overturned, there really seems no way of pursuing this further."

Now, however, there appeared to be a chance of Beth going home. A package consisting of several hours of district nursing each day and a rota of live-in assistants employed through direct payments which would cost £490 seemed to be a possibility. Beth was awaiting a community care reassessment by the newly unitary SSD covering the area where she owned her house.

Ian

Ian had severe Parkinson's disease. For five hours a day his body shook uncontrollably despite medication, but for many years his GP ignored the fact that Ian's wife needed help, despite letters to that effect from her GP.

"When you are dealing with things, when it's an everyday occurrence, you don't think that you're not coping very well, you just take each day as it comes. You can't see from the outside looking in that you're not coping. You are coping but you're going to pieces at the same time. And when you can't, you don't know the questions to ask, ie can I have a nurse? I think there should be some way, within some kind of practice or hospital, of people being given that information. You shouldn't have to go knocking on doors and saying can I have this, am I entitled to that? Someone should come out and say this is what you are entitled to, do you want it?" **(Ian's wife)**

Most of the community care literature that the couple had seen had been about elderly people or people with cancer, nothing relevant to a younger person with something like Parkinson's. Only a year ago, with a psychological crisis (a side-effect of a new medicine) and a change in consultant, had they been referred to social services. Four weeks' respite a year was offered plus 12 hours a week assistance from an agency. These hours

could not be in the evening, however, because this was the time that Ian regularly suffered his worst attacks. It was only after prolonged argument with the HA that a qualified nurse was provided for two evenings a week, but there continued to be a struggle to keep that provision. Recently, application to the ILF had resulted in an award that would cover 27 day hours a week and three nights. The couple were hoping that this might enable Ian to avoid respite care and possibly to go away on holiday with an assistant. (Author's note: stopping respite might reduce the LA's input below the ILF threshold.)

Parveen

Parveen was moving out of her parents' home into her own house and expecting to be offered direct payments, but there was a question mark over whether she needed turning during the night on the grounds of health or comfort. The HA had turned down a request for funding.

"Social services did try, but the health authority's argument is that, regardless of whether I got sores or not, I would still need turning because if I stuck to one level each night I am going to be uncomfortable. So the health authority have argued that it is not [its funding responsibility]."

Nora and Ken

Two years previously, Nora and Ken married and moved into the community after 20 years in residential care. Both needed a high level of community support, particularly Ken who had no effective motor capability below his neck and needed total assistance with all personal care. He was able to communicate his needs to people who knew him well with minimal speech and eye movements. The couple were funded for a joint package of assistance through the brokerage scheme. This enabled them to pay for personal assistants for each of them through the day-time and for Ken overnight. An application to the HA for funding for the overnight costs had been turned down and it was only by paying the assistants less than intended and negotiating with the ILF for use of its discretion around the £500 limit that a joint LA/ILF funding package could be agreed.

Unfortunately, it proved difficult to maintain Ken's package using direct employees because of the problem of finding suitable assistants who would provide the continuity necessary for someone with his level of need for the wages offered. It was decided that the only way his community support could succeed would be if an agency was employed. By the end of 1998 his care package was costing almost £1,000 a week, social services paying £611 towards this. A further application for a continuing care contribution from the HA towards this had failed.

Anna

Anna had advanced MS and no controlled movement in her arms, legs or feet. She was no longer able to eat or drink orally and had a gastrostomy tube. She was able to operate a possum with her tongue, which enabled her to control some aspects of her immediate environment and she wanted to remain in her own home. For this she had to be provided with a high-level support package consisting of a care brokerage payment of £390 a week (managed by Anna's cousin) to fund a live-in carer and three visits a day from in-house care workers to assist with transfers. The total cost put the package beyond the possibility of ILF support. A district nurse visited once a week and came in for the first two or three evenings of any new live-in care worker to ensure they managed the gastrostomy tube correctly, but medicines were administered by care workers. A submission for a continuing care contribution to the cost from the HA was turned down. One reason given was that the HA could not contribute to brokerage/ direct payments. The advantage to Anna of social services willingness to continue bearing all the costs was that she could continue to employ the people she wanted.

Case studies of people bridging the social/healthcare divide

Dan

By the end of 1998, Dan had a care package costing in total over £900. He paid £265 towards this from his own income (from an industrial injuries settlement) and the balance was divided between the LA and HA and the ILF. This package had been negotiated as a direct payment with funds transferred to social services from the HA. Part of the argument for continuing care funding had been that the care workers would be trained for and then provide physiotherapy.

Simon

Since leaving a Younger Disabled Unit a year previously, Simon had had a 24-hour package funded 50/50 by social services and the HA. He was not interested in the direct payments option, feeling that he had the flexibility and control he wanted from his existing arrangement with two local agencies. For £550 a week, these had been able to provide consistent workers whom Simon now saw as friends.

> *"They can cook, they are good company and I can ask for things to be done. My carers need to be able to drive and be over 25 for the insurance. I go to the bank, shopping, town, cinemas, restaurants, to see friends. I go out a few times each week."*

On top of the 50% HA funding, there was additional district nurse input from the health trust. The HA's perspective in this case was that its 50% funding was justified because the need for frequent catheter emptying and changing was beyond the input capacity of the mainstream district nurses, who were dealing with other health needs such as bowel care and medication. The social services perspective was that there was a range of quasi-nursing needs that overlapped with personal care and it was not cost-effective to make a rigid distinction in terms of who provided which. The HA had agreed to continue its funding beyond the initial six-month period after Simon's discharge, but subject to frequent review.

Frances

Frances paid for all her personal *and* healthcare needs with the combination of an ILF Extension Fund award of just over £400 a week and her DSS benefits (special transitional allowance of £198, DLA care component and Severe Disability Premium). Her care package in total cost £672. Social services had provided six hours a week of domestic help since she came out of residential care 13 years ago, but she had tried to have no more involvement with the department because of the experience that had originally led to her entering residential care. Frances used half of her money to pay for two self-employed assistants who covered various social care tasks and were on call at night and for emergencies, and the other half for 42 hours a week of qualified nursing assistance in the mornings and evenings.

> *"I need to have qualified people to handle me really because of my severe disability [her impairments were tetraplegia, asthma and visual impairment].... You have to know how to handle me and handle my equipment and to be able to react quickly if something goes wrong, if I need oxygen to be able to give it to me, to be able to give me my inhaler, my drugs and things like this. I can't read the bottles of drugs and it's really not acceptable for a carer to give me drugs they know nothing about. It's not fair on them insurance wise.... I need people to be aware of when I might need oxygen and to batter me a bit and say, don't you think you should have some. Also, they supply my catheter care, which would normally be provided by the health authority with their district nursing service. By having nurses do that role, it means that if my catheter comes out when they're getting me up, it can be replaced immediately. If I was relying on the NHS I'd have a carer get me up and then have to wait two or three hours for a district nurse to fit it. It would cost me more in*

> *care because I'd have to insist that the carer was with me waiting for the nurse to arrive. So it proves more cost-effective to have the qualified care most of the time. They can cope with any eventuality."*

Jacqueline

Jacqueline was generally very satisfied with the level of help she was getting through the Community MS Team (see the earlier example of effective working in Authority C).

> *"The [name of agency] look after me. They come in every morning, get me out of bed, washed, dressed, give me my breakfast and any medication I need, bring me downstairs and install me with all my necessary bits and pieces, so I can switch things on and also the care call button. That takes about an hour and a half. They come back at lunchtime and give me my lunch, empty my bag, install me in this chair with all my relevant bits and pieces around me and they come back at teatime, take me out of here into the kitchen and give me my tea and any medication I need, then bring me back in here. At about 9.45 they come back again and give me my medication for the night, undo all my gizmos, take me by chairlift and install me in bed, surrounded by the gizmos I need for the night. That goes on seven days a week, 365 days a year."*

In addition, a district nurse visited four mornings a week and once a night at 4am to turn her and give medication, and someone from another agency came for four hours each week to help with a variety of domestic tasks. Jacqueline went to physiotherapy sessions run by the MS Society in conjunction with the NHS every week and to hydrotherapy once a fortnight. If her husband had to be away overnight, there was enough money in the social services budget allocated to her to enable her to have a night sitter. She was also offered respite care for up to five weeks a year. Jacqueline realised that she received a high level of assistance and praised the MS Team highly: "From my point of view it works beautifully well."

Apart from the above examples from our interviewee sample, the ILFs, as mentioned in Chapter 4, have a number of clients whose total care packages can be supported at a cost well above £500 a week because of a HA contribution. Some of these packages exceed £1,000.

Summary

People with high support needs have very different outcomes in different areas according to how continuing care criteria are applied.

NHS financial support for services in the grey area where social and healthcare responsibilities continue to be debated can allow someone with needs assessed by social services as costing more than £500 to access the assistance they need rather than have to go into residential care. One reason for this is that the expenditure ceiling set by the ILF does not take account of HA funding.

Even where there is a strategic acknowledgement of the need for a flexible approach to joint funding, the structures often inhibit creative, best value solutions. Apart from jealously guarded budgets and professional roles, two other barriers are also presented: (i) social care is subject to charges whereas NHS provision is not, and (ii) the NHS is unable to use its resources to fund direct payments. Examples, however, show that these barriers are not insurmountable and the introduction of direct payments in particular can successfully challenge current rigidities.

Physiotherapy is one area where many disabled people feel they are getting inadequate support but where personal assistants can be trained to help.

8
Independent living

Independent living is not just about living in the community rather than in residential care, but about the quality of that life and the extent to which disabled people achieve choices that non-disabled people take for granted. Our research into the circumstances of people with high support needs revealed the compromises that are made, sometimes as a result of resource limitations, sometimes as a result of the structures of funder and provider organisations and the attitudes of staff within them.

Residential care

Among our interviewees were 14 who had lived in residential care for at least two years of their lives and two others who had failed in their attempts to move from residential care out into the community. One of the latter, **Beth**, whose situation was described in Chapter 5, was the victim of disputed responsibility between social services and the HA. An application to the ILF 93 Fund several years previously had been withdrawn pending the outcome of that negotiation but she was still in the home. The other person we interviewed in residential care had been the subject of an argument about funding responsibility between three different LAs with no satisfactory outcome for him. The assessed cost of a community care package for him would have been well above the ILF 93 Fund limit.

Both of these people had a fierce desire to live in the community and, whatever other factors might have been involved in each of their cases, appeared to have no greater personal care and health needs than many of the others we interviewed.

In our discussions with social services and voluntary sector staff in the six authorities, there was a widespread view that there were physically disabled people in residential care who *could* be in the community and that many of these were in inappropriate nursing home places rather than in the more expensive homes which catered for the younger age range.

> *"It's a nightmare trying to negotiate anything above bog standard nursing homes. We used to be able to get people into external high-quality nursing home places, but not now."* (**Social worker**)

Even where there were young disabled person's units and these cost less than £500, there were often reservations on the part of social workers about the level and appropriateness of the social activity they offered.

Some of the disabled people we talked with, who had moved out of residential care, spoke of others they had left behind who wanted to leave. One local voluntary organisation run by disabled people had tried to make contact with people in care to talk about opportunities for independent living, but felt that they had been blocked at every turn. It was important, they felt, that people were given the opportunity to know what was possible, otherwise only the most determined were able to challenge professional gatekeeping.

> *"I was about 22. I then got into the NHS and ended up in a young disabled unit. Not of my choosing but I was told that it was either there or a geriatric hospital. So I hadn't got any choice in the matter. I always said all along that I wanted to live on my own and be independent, but social services, when I was about 18, wouldn't believe it was possible, so it just never happened.... My goals were to live in a flat of my own, go to university and go to work. My GP used to call it pipe dreams*

*and nobody believed it was ever going to be possible." (**Frances**, who eventually achieved the first two of those goals with the help of an ILF Extension Fund award)*

Unlike resettlement programmes for people with learning disabilities, where there was HA funding, there was no pot of money to bring people with physical disabilities into the community and, for people who had been in residential care for a long time, there was little financial incentive for doing so. One SSD had made efforts to convey to voluntary organisations running residential homes that it could not be expected to pick up the costs of people transferred into the community with high support needs. It was concerned about one particular case where it had not been consulted over a package that would cost more than £600 a week.

In Authority E, all residential placements for younger disabled people were out-of-area. Some of these people had expressed a desire to move into the community, but often this had not been pursued beyond the initial expression of interest, one reason given being their lack of roots in the area. However, a small number had succeeded. After initially refusing because their placements had been funded by other authorities, this SSD had recently agreed to cover the community care costs of four people coming out of private or voluntary sector institutions located within its own boundaries. Two of these were among the people we interviewed.

Nora and **Ken** had been in residential care in Authority E for 29 and 27 years respectively. When they decided that they wanted to marry and be housed locally, the authority initially refused to take on this responsibility because their placements had been funded by two other LAs. Recently, however, Authority E's previous ruling that it would not rehouse and support people in their position had been overturned and the couple moved out.

"Moving out into a community is not just moving out and getting someone to care for you. It's your social life, your friends you've made around you, the places you like to go, the whole network. Losing them and the choice of a place to live in, to go back to your old boroughs is not the ideal thing."(Nora)

There were, of course, many examples among our interviewees of people fighting to remain in the community rather than go into residential care.

*"There is no way I'm going to be institutionalised, no way. I want my life. There are lots of people worse off than me. But I am me, no one else, and it's my view that if I live on my own as much as I can and try and do as much as I can, then I'm still living. I think there's a line between the two. I would rather try and live than just exist. To me a residential home is just an existence. I live a humdrum life now, but I'm independent. I do as much as I can." (**Mike**)*

There were also examples which point up the need for professionals to encourage disabled people to attempt independent living and avoid residential care:

*"Basically I didn't decide [to move out of her parents' house]. I was under pressure from my consultant to move on and go independent, because he'd known me since I had the transverse myalitus and hence the disability, and he thought it was about time that I went independent. It was pointed out to me as well from my social worker that if I didn't go independent and something happened to either my mum or dad, then I would have to go into a home. One of my ex-social workers came across this flat and put my name forward. But it was not through my choice.... Now I've moved into a place of my own, I wouldn't have it any other way. I love the independence. I find it a good challenge and very stimulating. I feel like a normal person." (**Laura**)*

Housing

A prerequisite for independent living for people with high support needs is the sort of housing that minimises the extent to which the assistance of other people is necessary and makes that assistance as easy to deliver as possible. Many of the people in our study found that this was extremely difficult to secure.

One reason was the scarcity of suitable buildings. People required space not just for themselves and their wheelchairs, but for their assistants as well. Where night-time cover was needed this meant an extra bedroom. When contemplating a move, someone with a deteriorating condition would have to anticipate the time when this might be the situation, but two-bedroomed flats or bungalows for rent to single disabled people were hard to find; in some areas it was seemingly impossible. A disabled parent with a young child among our interviewees described the difficulty of persuading the LA of her need for a property which would make it easier for her to care for her child rather than depend totally upon other people to care for both of them.

Some of those who moved out of residential care or a parent's home felt that their desire for a home of their own had been given low priority by housing authorities. **Samantha** had needed 24-hour care when she left residential care:

> "I'd been awarded the ILF money for about a year before and I got so worried because I kept getting letters from them saying that unless you can start utilising the funding that's been allocated to you we will have to reconsider you and reassess you. So I was getting absolutely panic-stricken.... I explained that I would have to have a two- or three-bedroomed place, preferably three bedroomed because I need storage space for spare wheelchairs and a hoist, etc. They kept offering me one-bedroomed flats in multi-storey flats in the most horrendous areas of [name of authority] and I had to keep turning them down."

Other interviewees also had the experience of being offered, or having to stay in, houses in rough areas where they were hassled by neighbours or found it difficult to recruit assistants, particularly when those assistants had to visit after dark. A few were living in accommodation that was totally unsuitable:

> "I don't go out. It's too difficult to get down the stairs.... The truth is unless I change my home, there's very little the occupational therapist can do to help. We've discussed a lift, but even if I had one, there are still some very steep steps outside the flat. The gradient would have to be very low for me to negotiate it in my wheelchair and in order to do that the ramp would have to reach to the other side of the road, so I'm stuck. The only thing I can do is move flats ... to one with a palatial bathroom. As far as I'm concerned the kitchen can be small as hell, but I need a big bathroom!" **(Mohammed)**

Mohammed's assistants currently had great difficulty helping him bathe because the bathroom was too small to allow a hoist to be used.

There were usually long waiting lists for adaptations. Also some of those who had moved into specially adapted properties had found that the adaptations were inappropriate. **Nora** found that she was not able to use her cooker because of its position:

> "So my cooking is now come to instructing.... You gain your independence and then something like that happens and you lose it."

Two people who had closely overseen the work being done on houses being prepared for them stressed the importance of being involved at that stage. It took **Ahmed**, who was leaving his parents' home, four years and a protracted wrangle with a housing association to find a suitable house and to get the adaptations he felt he needed. When visiting while work was being done, he had found that surfaces were being put in at the wrong height, and many other things that would make a significant difference to his ability to be independent also needed correction.

Brian, who had enough money to buy a house but not to have the necessary adaptations carried out, found himself in a frustrating situation because of another waiting list:

> *"The rules seemed to be very badly thought through. You couldn't apply for a Home Improvement Grant until you were the title holder of the property you wanted it done on. But the waiting list for a grant was anything up to two years. So I was faced with the possibility of buying somewhere that I couldn't live in for two years, which seemed totally ridiculous to me."*

Social activities

In the six authorities we visited, social services policy and practice relating to the promotion of social activity for severely disabled people lacked consistency. Although specialist social workers claimed always to try to take social needs into account, arguing social isolation or stretching times assessed for personal care tasks, there was a widespread feeling that "The arguments against funding social activities for elderly people are increasingly being used for younger physically disabled people in a way they never used to be" (social worker). Even more than the provision of health or personal care, this was resource led, the icing on the cake of basic community care. People with only physical impairments were less likely to be funded for their participation in social activities than people with challenging behaviour, especially where such funding would come on top of a high level of assistance for personal care.

There were, however, some encouraging signs. In Authority F, for example, there had previously been very strict gatekeeping by social services, limiting funding to personal care tasks, but the new unitary authority had explicitly adopted the

social model of disability as a guiding principle and there was hope among some care managers of a significant cultural shift in the direction of more explicit support for social activity. They were currently 'testing out waters' with their team leaders.

In this authority, as in others, direct payments were opening the door to support for social activity. Part of this was to do with the very principles that direct payments were based upon. It was generally acknowledged that direct payments were about people managing their own lives and that people with such an 'independent' attitude would expect more from community care than merely enough help to get up in the morning, go to bed at night and be assisted with eating and getting to the toilet in between.

> *"**Barbara** is currently in dispute with social services over her request for extra hours.... She explained that she wanted the extra hours so that she could go out in the evenings. She attends meetings and also likes to go out socially. She has personal care needs when out because she cannot transfer in and out of the car without help and also needs help to use the toilet. On nights when she is at home she needs help with toileting and her son has to assist her, but he also likes to go out. Social services do not take account of social care needs even when there are personal care needs, hence the dispute." (ILF **Visiting Social Worker report**)*

In Authority F, it was suggested that, although care managers did not generally highlight social activities in their assessments (one team leader said that she deleted any reference to social hours in any assessment that came to her), a high proportion of the people on direct payments probably had an element of this in their care packages.

For someone already getting more than £200 a week from social services, the extra funding that would facilitate social activity was often more easily secured from the ILF. But getting funding from the ILF for assistants to be with the disabled person outside their home still had to be justified on the basis of need for personal care during that time.

Gillian recognised that getting her support package over the £200 threshold was significant and had complained about her social services level of assessment:

> *"The idea is that if your care package goes over £200, that's when you can apply to the ILF. We were near to the £200 but not quite there. We needed a few extra hours from social services."*

Eventually Gillian was successful in pressing her case and her application to the ILF gave her 40 extra hours a week.

Sarah and her husband had been able to organise a much more satisfactory arrangement through direct payments than through the previous agency contract:

> *"We have two hours in the week 'social time' to allow either Sarah or myself to take the children out, so we spend time with the children, and we have nine hours at the weekend for social time.... For example, if Sarah wants to go out, say to the pictures on a Friday night, or to the pub, she's got a carer who can take her. I look after the children while she goes out, or if I want to go out, we take it in turns. We would go out together but they're not there for babysitting, only to look after the disabled person." (Sarah's husband)*

This was an important achievement for the couple, who had been arguing for a long time that the LA should be supporting Sarah in her parenting responsibility. As well as introducing some flexibility into how community care money was used, it seemed that new direct payments arrangements might also have the potential to be

of more help to disabled parents by eroding the rigid distinctions between adult care and child protection represented by the two separate LA budgets.

As well as the greater likelihood of having some element of funding for social activity agreed, compared with the limitations with traditional services, direct payments could be a better arrangement for recruiting employees for this purpose, because personal choice of such assistants could be crucial. For **Dora**, for example, it was important to employ someone who shared her interests and was from her own Afro-Caribbean culture:

> *"Compared to what I had before, I'm a lot more satisfied. The care brokerage system is fantastic.... I have the privilege of choice. I can get carers who I think can help me culturally which is important to me. The type of food I want to have, getting my hair shampooed, going to church with me...."*

If someone was getting help from the ILF Extension Fund, where the upper limit on awards was £560 rather than £300, the potential for getting assistance for hours that would cover social activity was greater. **Robert** had an Extension Fund award of £445 a week, which, together with social services funding of £161 (not a direct payment), covered three sleepovers and 61 day hours from an agency. He lived with his mother who was in her late sixties and found that the help he was able to pay for, enhanced by the purchase of a car insured for any driver and a car hoist, gave him the independence he wanted to go out to the pub with people of his own age as well as further afield during the day.

> *"Although Robert's condition has deteriorated since I visited the first time six years ago, it is quite amazing to see the difference which ILF help has made. Both Robert and his mother are thriving on the care they are now able to purchase. From a house which was sad and silent, there is*

*now a lot of coming and going and this is stimulating. The quality of the care they have been able to purchase is very high." (**ILF visiting social worker**)*

By contrast, in a different authority, another young man was getting very unsatisfactory provision for help with social activities. He attended a day centre three times a week where everyone else was much older, and he was in respite care for seven weeks a year in a similar environment. **Jim** had had an ILF Extension Fund award of just £25 a week since 1990 and was only now thinking of asking for more (until recently it had not been possible to get an increase in an Extension Fund award unless there had been a significant increase in personal care needs). He and his mother were also thinking about direct payments.

> *"He says to me, 'Mum, they're lovely people and they love me to bits and I get on well with everybody, but I've got nothing in common with old people'. This has been the problem from day one, they don't cater for young people.... We've even asked that perhaps somebody, a carer, could come and take Jim out, but it's just not done.... He'd like to have his own place basically with full care. That's what we'd all like, for Jim to have a life. At the moment, though we do have some care at home, Jim has no social life. This is not the life he wants." (**Jim's mother**)*

Many of our interviewees yearned for some extra funding that would give them the flexibility to use their care assistants for social activities:

> *"I'd like to go out on the days when I'm not on dialysis. You get rather blue when you're in the house all the time. I mean it would be a delight to go to the shops or go.... Gosh, I think it would be my birthday if I went out and did a bit of shopping or looked round Marks and Spencer. It's things like that you miss, you really do miss those things. But there aren't enough hours. Anyway you*

*can't use your Independent Living like that. You can't use it to go out." (**Jane**)*

There were others among our interviewees who also thought that ILF awards could not be used for going out, but some used them for that purpose whenever possible.

> *"The agency used to get me up on a Sunday but, starting this Sunday gone, the district nurses are getting me up on a Sunday. So that's saving me some money in order to go out a bit more. That's what I need, I need to get out. So that money then can go towards actual quality time.... When I first went into a chair, there was nowhere that was wheelchair accessible. You couldn't go to the cinema. But now you can go basically anywhere." (**Jenny**)*

One additional limitation upon social activities with personal assistants, however, was that the cost of extra tickets and meals out for them sometimes had to be found.

Mike said that he had been allowed some weekend care because his children, who lived with their mother, came to visit him and this enabled him to go out with them. He did not know how long this would continue and whether, when the children were older, he would lose these hours.

> *"My weekend carer is allowed to take me out. If that was to stop I'd be existing, not living, because I'd be seven days a week stuck in here.... If my weekend money was to stop when the children are a certain age.... It's really worrying me. If [name of authority] has tight limits on their money, who could I get to fund me for this? Would the ILF fund me or would someone else?"*

Day centres
Where people are provided with a place at a LA day centre for four or five days a week, the ILF 93 Fund threshold of £200 can very often be

reached. (It was even suggested that day centre costings might sometimes be deliberately tailored to the ILF requirement of £40 a day!) This then makes it possible to apply for an ILF award which can be used to pay for additional social care needs. However, it is more likely that people with severe learning disabilities will be offered such a high level of day centre provision than people with physical impairments, many of whom would not consider such a service appropriate anyway.

Jim (see above) was an example of someone for whom available day centre provision was inappropriate. He was getting additional funding from the ILF Extension Fund which was not contingent upon a certain level of social services input so, if he had wanted to, he could have withdrawn from the day centre without losing his ILF award. This would not have been the case for people getting 93 Fund awards.

Gillian's social worker said that the £74 a week day centre element of her package would probably fund an extra 12 to 14 hours. He thought that the implications of the ILF threshold would be recognised but whether the resources would be there to offer or not was another matter.

There had been consultations in Authority D about changing day centre services to other day activities which would be attractive for younger disabled people, but there were fears that the latter would prove more expensive.

Some of our interviewees who had day centre provision spoke of cutbacks in availability, others about the quality of what was offered there. **Mike** felt that the users of his day centre had become more passive. There were no longer outings and it was more difficult to get physiotherapy.

"They spent a lot of money decorating, which we moaned about. We would rather have the money put towards transport to go out. Now it's more of a hospice and I feel sorry for the people who go

there. You get more and more people who just sit and do nothing."

When Mike withdrew from his day centre, his package was reviewed, but he was not provided with replacement assistance at home and the ILF would not cover what was seen as a social services reduction.

Respite care

The term respite was used in two ways: one meant giving informal carers a break from their normal routine, the other meant giving the disabled person a holiday. Although some of our interviewees had the opportunity to go to places that they liked, traditional respite in a residential or nursing home was often the only sort of break offered and was not what they wanted. They would be with much older people, for instance, and would not be taken out at all.

*"Whenever they've offered **Sarah** respite, it's in a home and she doesn't want to go. She's a young woman, she wants to be able to go somewhere that she's got a carer to go with her. So we said to her social worker, Sarah wants respite but she wants to go to a proper holiday resort that accommodates disabled people. It took them about four weeks and they had a meeting with their legal department, but they did it." (**Sarah's husband**, who stayed at home with the children)*

*"It's a bit of flexibility. It's really good that social services were able to look at the problems and say yes. What do I want to go and pay residential for. I've got young personal assistants and one of them came to Blackpool with me. I had a proper holiday." (**Sarah**)*

Care management

The inability of social workers to provide adequate ongoing support was reflected in the comments of several interviewees in one authority:

"There's not enough people to go and check people and see what their needs are, if they'd improved or worsened. If you had that, you'd have a record, but they're not keeping records. Quite frankly it's just a 'don't care' attitude." (Elisabeth)

"I'd like someone that comes and looks and says, look that isn't quite right, leave that alone, do this, don't do that, and I will come and sort it out for you. Somebody that oversees something. A social worker used to be able to do this for me. She used to write letters for me and took a lot of the hassle and burden off me. But then she upped and left.... I want someone to come along and give me some good, sound, positive advice." (Len's mother)

Elsewhere, many people were content just to know that they had a reliable contact in the department.

"About every couple of months, he rings up and asks if everything is alright and I say yes. That's the main thing. We are left alone so I can deal with things." (Sarah)

It was the variation and high turnover of social workers that others found frustrating:

"The first one really knew what he was on about but the one I've got now doesn't. You'd think she would know ways and things to do but she doesn't seem to have an idea.... Some are good, some are bad, some are indifferent. If you talk to them and they're obviously not listening to you, you just feel you're banging your head against a brick wall and wasting your time and theirs probably." (Dave)

"I spoke to the duty officer last Friday. They said they were going to ring me back on Monday, but nobody did, they never do, that happens a lot." (Mike)

The familiarity of individual social workers with the circumstances and concerns of younger disabled people, as opposed to the much greater

number of older people in their caseloads, could be significant. In Authority B we were told that there were six social workers who had originally been in a specialist team and were now scattered throughout the department. Younger disabled people tended to be allocated to them:

"Our colleagues back off. Disabled people are seen as stroppy individuals who know what they want!" (Social worker)

There was praise for the specialist disability team in Authority C:

"The social services at [name of local office] are marvellous. You could speak to anyone in their office and they all understand what you're saying and if they can't help in any way they will find some person who can help. They are not the kind of social workers that in the past you wouldn't want in your house, you know, who came in and told you what they thought. They don't tell you what they can do, they listen to you." (Ian's wife)

Many of our interviewees received some form of direct payments (LA or ILF) and handled their own care management. Because of their different personalities and abilities and the availability of supportive family and friends, they had a wide range of need for outside help with this. At one end of the spectrum **Ahmed** did not find his social services reviews at all useful:

"It's good to sort of keep a social worker doing a job, but I don't find it that useful really. I just have to tell a social worker that everything's okay. Because you're in control of it you seem to be able to find solutions to problems for yourself. Before, when it was controlled by the social worker, he was the problem solver.... My social worker's very flexible, but even he finds [the new arrangement] very challenging. I think he's from the old school of social workers where his job was to solve problems for disabled people. Sometimes I find that very limiting, you know that disabled people

are sort of the caseloads of social workers.... I think social services departments need to change their philosophy and the way they manage their care provision in a more creative way, a more flexible way than set hours and set agencies and such. They need to look at the client as a human being rather than just a person who needs personal care, an all round person. What are their needs, what do they want to do with their lives? Imagination!"

At the other end of the spectrum were people who found their social workers, or the support services set up in conjunction with direct payments, invaluable.

"I did the interviewing with support because, although the person who was supporting me said during my latter interviews they didn't know why they were there because I seemed to be able to do it very well, it's just nice to have someone there." **(Pat)**

Issues around direct payments have been described to some extent in Chapter 6 and are the subject of other research and a Department of Health review (see Chapter 2), so they will not be discussed in detail here. But it is worth noting that, although some people in our research preferred not to take on the extra responsibilities involved, those who *were* getting direct payments described the outcome for them positively in terms of choice, control, dignity and direction. The comments of **Hilary** and **Doreen** below illustrate some of these feelings:

"Flexibility, choice, independence. It gives everything that the other packages [in-house Homecare, then private agency] didn't give. You don't have to go through the third degree to get rid of somebody. I mean Jenny was late for three mornings. She blamed it on her alarm clock, she blamed it on her fella, she blamed it on a leak. I don't know whether there's truth in any of it, but I said 'Listen, you're late again and I'm cutting your

hours down and giving them to someone else.' I told her straight and she hasn't been late since. Now, I couldn't have said that to social services carers, I couldn't even have said it to an agency carer, because they arrange their times with social services. But with direct payments I can do that. I know what I want and I know how I want it." **(Hilary)**

"We get to say who, what, why and when, and that alone means so much. It's not so much being the boss over other people, it's being boss of your own life again. You're not answerable to other people, you're answerable to yourself, and other people are then answerable to you.... Now I can say 'Well, I want a bath now', 'Come on, let's go and do it', 'I would like this done'. 'Right we'll do it.' 'I want to go to such and such a place.' 'Right, no problem. We'll phone a taxi.' It's about having that control again, you being the boss of your own life." **(Doreen)**

Several interviewees stressed how important direct payments had been in changing the nature of the support they received to help them in their roles as parents. Previously, rigid distinctions between personal care and childcare had limited the effectiveness of social services support.

Apart from issues about direct payments revealed in earlier chapters, such as the problem of getting HA funding, it is also worth mentioning briefly two other concerns raised by a number of interviewees about how direct payments systems operated. The first of these was that it was important to people, particularly those with variable conditions, that they had the freedom to use their allocated hours as flexibly as possible. Having a contingency budget was also valuable because it gave people a sense of security that they could cope with the emergencies that very often occurred for people with high support needs. This was something that was offered with some social services schemes but not by the ILF. The second, related, concern was that the record-keeping requirements of some LAs were unnecessarily burdensome, even after packages had been established for several years. This rigidity undermined the flexibility and autonomy that should underpin independent living arrangements. In the words of **Samantha**:

> *"I break all the rules, I'm sure I do. But it's not as if the money is being spent on things that it isn't intended for. Yes, some weeks there's money left over but I save for when I want to go on holiday and I'm going to need a lot of extra cover. Sometimes I have to take two people away with me so you know I have to pay two people's wages. It worries me that I do that, I break the rules.... I mean it's not as if you could live the high life on the money because, if you haven't got somebody here, you don't get out of bed."*

One thing that marred the experience of independent living for some of our interviewees was their lack of security about future support. Sometimes there was a fear of cutbacks, sometimes an awareness that extra funding would not be available if their care needs increased or agency rates rose.

> *"You hear of so many cutbacks you begin to wonder if they will start saying you have to have a smaller package. It's like they're playing God with your life. You've just got independence but you don't feel a hundred per cent. There's always this nagging feeling at the back of your mind."* **(Gillian)**

> *"I asked the social worker about what happens if I needed extra in the future and she said, well you won't be allowed any extra hours. But I've got MS and with that condition the chances are I'm going to deteriorate at some stage in the future and I don't know what will happen when I do need extra care."* **(Pauline)**

The age divide

People over 65 are disadvantaged in a number of ways: they cannot get help from the ILF (except for some fortunate ones who were accepted by the original pre-1993 Fund and are now clients of the Extension Fund); they have not been able to access LA direct payments (the extent to which this is likely to change as a result of the policy change revealed in the 1998 Department of Health White Paper remains to be seen); and they are categorised as 'elderly' or 'older people' rather than 'disabled', which usually means lower or more rigid ceilings on LA community care expenditure (see Chapter 5).

As described in Chapter 3, three of our six SSDs had specialist physical disability teams which operated separately from teams for older people (that is, over 65), but there were some differences in how this separation worked. In Authority A, for example, clients were handed over from one team to the other as they reached 65. Disability team care managers would attempt to get packages set up and "watertight" before the changeover, in the expectation that this provision would not be reduced unless there was a drastic change in care needs. In Authority E, by contrast, clients would stay with the disability team.

In general, differences in willingness to fund the older and younger age groups tended to reflect differences in residential or nursing home costs and the relative unwillingness of LAs to top up fees for over-65s. The situation in Authority E, described by one of its care managers in a letter to the researcher, illustrates some of the issues around this:

> *"The physical disability team (which takes referrals up to 65) operates on a more flexible basis. Although the teams technically share the same eligibility criteria, people tend to be offered more care. This is partly due to the philosophy of promoting independence. People on the Physical*

Disability Team are more likely to be able to go shopping with their carers if they choose to do so, whereas, for the over 65 team this is not allowed (ie no extra time would be allowed to make this possible). It is also related to the vast difference in the cost of residential care between the divisions. The Physical Disability Team could expect to pay £750 for residential care. It is therefore more economical to support people at home, with care arrangements costing more than £225 per week. We can of course access different funding channels for this client group as well, ie ILF. People also tend to be more vocal and there are fewer clients to support."

Compared with the high-level packages available to people under-65, the most community care that an over 65 could hope for would be three visits a day for help with meals and getting to the toilet and maybe a couple of hours of cleaning. No live-in or night care would be available. An example was given of a man of 69 with MS and a heart condition whose wife was his main carer. There was currently a discussion at management level about whether or not he should be allowed to revert to the Disability Team. The implications for the man were significant. Under the rules of the Physical Disability Team he would be able to get four weeks' respite a year in a specialist MS home. Under the Elderly Persons' Team, he would be restricted to one week in a council residential home for elderly people. Another example was of a woman with MS who lived alone and was referred at the age of 62. She was able to get direct payments. Three years older and she would not have been eligible for these and would not have been able to go outside her house with a personal assistant. She might instead have been offered a place at a day centre.

For the budget-holding managers within the department, there were inevitably debates around these issues. Should, for example, the physical disability budget be expected to pay for extra care for the age-related deterioration of someone with a longer-standing disability?

Summary

There are some people in residential care against their will because of a failure of social services and HAs to agree the funding for community care. Others are there because different LAs dispute their responsibility for funding.

There are also worrying indications that people are placed in inappropriate nursing homes because of LA budget constraints. Social workers make attempts to maintain people in the community within limited budgets for as long as possible, but unless community care can be provided at a cheaper price there is a financial disincentive involved which becomes more powerful in the context of tighter budgets.

A prerequisite for independent living for people with high support needs is housing that minimises the extent to which the assistance of other people is necessary and makes that assistance as easy to deliver as possible. This often means extra rooms to accommodate personal assistants and equipment, as well as adaptations that suit varying individual requirements. A scarcity of suitable properties in suitable locations, waiting lists for adaptations and lack of involvement of the disabled people themselves in designing the environments they need make this extremely difficult to secure.

Two contradictory trends affect the funding of support for disabled people's social activity. One is the contraction of services, which means that funding for anything other than securing a person's safety in their own home is being squeezed out. The other is that direct payments packages are opening up opportunities for social activity through their flexibility and their acknowledgement of disabled people's aspirations for independent living.

The ILF has often been the only means by which people with high support needs have accessed enough funding for personal care to be able to use it flexibly and thereby support social activity, but getting the required £200 worth of support from social services to open this door can sometimes be easier for people with learning disabilities who attend day centres all week than for people with physical impairments for whom day centre provision is unattractive. Some people with ILF Extension Fund awards, where the ceiling is £560 (in addition to any social services input), have the greatest potential.

Respite, which offers carers a break from their normal routine but which also gives disabled people the opportunity of a proper holiday rather than a spell in inappropriate residential care, seems to be desirable but unusual.

People have varying levels of need for professional care management, but the minimum requirement of a consistent and reliable contact within social services is not always available. Specialist physical disability social workers are valued for their knowledge, as are well-resourced direct payments support services for their encouragement and support. At the other end of the spectrum, communication channels are poor and direct payments are badly resourced and supported.

Disabled people over 65 are categorised as 'elderly' or 'older people' which usually means lower ceilings on community care expenditure and more rigidity in the application of those ceilings. They have not been able to get top-up funding from the ILF since 1993 or to access LA direct payments. The government has announced its intention of making the latter a legal possibility in the near future, but it remains to be seen, on the one hand, the extent to which LAs will encourage this option and, on the other, the demand that will be generated as older people, and perhaps more significantly their carers, become aware of the possibility.

9
Conclusions

One result of our research has been the demonstration of some of the ways in which people with high support needs are forced to compromise their aspirations for independent living in order to comply with resource-driven services. But the study also revealed important developments which have widened many people's options. Where there has been a move away from social services' rigid use of in-house services, for example, or direct payments have been promoted with enthusiasm, it has been possible to offer much more user choice and control, leading to better qualitative outcomes.

The problem is that there is now a growing tension between raised expectations and ever-tightening constraints on expenditure. There are also wide discrepancies between the outcomes for people with similarly high needs depending on where they live and when their support packages were set up. The £500 ceiling operated by the ILF 93 Fund on the packages of care it supports jointly with LAs and the fact that this ceiling has remained unchanged since 1993, as has the Fund's own maximum award of £300, have constrained the potential some people with high support needs might otherwise have to achieve independent living. The ILF limits reinforce the tendency of LAs to impose rigid cost ceilings of their own to cope with budget pressures, rather than seek more creative and flexible answers to disabled people's aspirations. It is arguable that, with the Best Value framework now in place in LAs, there should be no need for limits of this kind at all.

Putting choice and control, together with fairness, at the heart of service objectives is clearly a difficult challenge for social care managers with inadequate budgets. But there must be better ways of using resources for people with high support needs than some of the current arrangements described in this report. Indeed, other packages of assistance are described which show what might be possible when user-defined outcomes are given priority over traditional practices and service provider boundaries. The difference can be between staying in the community and having to enter residential care, or between having assistance that is responsive to the choice of the user and assistance that is a complex patchwork of provision determined by professional roles and timetables.

When the constraints on resources are viewed as less than paramount, it is clear that, far from disabled people 'asking for too much', many are asking for too little. What is required is a framework for diversity that enables users and social services assessors to work out the most effective arrangement of support while paying adequate attention to quality of life values such as how individuals view their needs for privacy and for social interaction as well as for their own home in the community. The range of options currently presented to users is often very narrow. Resources are locked into provision such as day centres and patterns of short visits which, though suiting some people, are inappropriate to many others.

For people with physical impairments, the consequences of separate budgets and restrictive practices can themselves be disabling. For those with high support needs, the mismatch between social and health policies in terms of direct payments and independent living is of particular concern. It is to be hoped that the practical realisation of the various partnerships encouraged in recent government initiatives will have a positive impact on social health needs, with the values of independent living at the centre of any future development.

As a direct outcome of this research and a contribution to that development, various questions are raised for policy makers and practitioners, both nationally and locally. Here are some of the key ones:

- Are any disabled people living unwillingly in residential care? Have they been identified and have *all* possibilities, including direct payments, been explored to help them live and be active in the community?

- Are disabled people's needs for social contact and for activity outside their homes assessed and provided for or, at the very least, acknowledged and recorded if resources are not currently available to satisfy them?

- Is the ILF 93 Fund being used to full effect? Are all social workers and managers working with disabled people aware of how a social services input of £200 worth of services to someone who meets the Fund's criteria can open the door to greater opportunities for independent living?

- Do 'respite' arrangements offer what disabled people themselves, as well as their carers, want and are care managers fully aware of the variety of facilities that may be used?

- Do support packages allow people flexibility to have services at the times they want them and, within reason, to change those times to suit themselves? Do those services adequately respect people's desire for privacy?

- Do commissioning specifications ensure that only empowering service providers are awarded contracts and do disabled people get the opportunity for a full annual review of their community care packages?

- How will new partnerships between social and health services facilitate user-centred decision making where care costs are high? Will it be possible, for example, for NHS funds in joint budgets, or individual packages, to support direct payments?

- Is there recognition of ways in which personal assistants may be trained to support health provision such as physiotherapy?

- How will overall funding, including ILF maximums, respond to upward pressures due to inflation, Working Time Regulations and lifting restrictions?

- Should the £500 ceiling operated by the ILF be raised, or abandoned altogether, leaving it up to LAs to decide whether certain cases merit spending more than £200 a week?

- Where a low demand for direct payments reflects negative attitudes of social services staff, how can this resistance be overcome? Are low budgets for direct payments and unnecessarily tight criteria in effect constraining the promotion of this option?

- Are organisations of disabled people being encouraged and funded to set up personal assistance support schemes? More generally, is the expertise of disabled people in this area being acknowledged and harnessed?

- Are services provided on the basis of ability to benefit from them? To what extent are over-65s unfairly excluded from independent living opportunities presented to under-65s?

- Is there a case for a National Service Framework for people with physical impairments which, among other things, would promote national equity in terms of opportunities for independent living?

References

Audit Commission (1997) *The coming of age: Improving care services for older people*, London: Audit Commission.

Bennett, F. (1996) *Highly charged: Policy issues surrounding charging for non-residential care*, York: Joseph Rowntree Foundation.

Craig, G. (1993) *The community care reforms and local government change*, Social Research Paper No 1, Humberside: University of Humberside.

Davis, A., Ellis, K. and Rummery, K. (1997) *Access to assessment: Perspectives of practitioners, disabled people and carers*, Bristol: The Policy Press.

DoH (Department of Health) (1994) Letter to Director of Berkshire Social Services, 1 September.

DoH (1995) *NHS responsibilities for meeting continuing care needs*, HSG (95), London: DoH.

DoH (1997a) *The new NHS: Modern, dependable*, London: HMSO.

DoH (1997b) *Community Care (Direct Payments) Act 1996: Policy and practice guidance*, London: HMSO.

DoH (1998) *Modernising social services*, DoH White Paper, London: HMSO.

Hardy, B. (1998) *Report of 1997 survey of UKHCA members*, Leeds: Nuffield Institute for Health.

Hasler, F., Campbell, J. and Zarb, G. (1999) *Direct routes to independence: A guide to local authority implementation and management of direct payments*, London: Policy Studies Institute.

House of Commons Select Health Committee (1999) *Relationship between health and social services*, London: HMSO.

Independent Living Funds (1998) *Annual Report*, Nottingham.

Kestenbaum, A. (1996) *An opportunity lost: Social services use of the Independent Living Transfer*, The Disablement Income Group.

Kestenbaum, A. (1997) *Disability-related costs and charges for community care*, The Disablement Income Group.

Laing & Buisson Ltd (1998a) *The homecare market 1998*, Laing & Buisson.

Laing & Buisson Ltd (1998b) *Community Care Market News*, October.

Royal Commission on Long Term Care (1999) *With respect to old age: Long term care – rights and responsibilities*, London: The Sationery Office.

Zarb, G. and Nadash, P. (1994) *Cashing in on independence: Comparing the costs and benefits of cash and services*, British Council of Organisations of Disabled People.

Appendix A: Independent Living 93 Fund eligibility criteria

The Trust Deed of the 93 Fund determines who is eligible for its help. A successful applicant must meet *all* of the following criteria:

- be at least 16 and under 66 years of age;

- receive the highest care component of the Disability Living Allowance* *and* be able to live in the community for at least the next six months;

- have capital of less than £8,000 *and* an income that is insufficient to cover the cost of the care needed;

- be assessed by the LA as being at risk of entering residential care, or capable of leaving it to live in the community, *and* receive at least £200 worth of services per week from the LA (net of any charge) *and* be assessed as needing additional care. The 93 Fund is able to pay up to a maximum of £300 per week.

Note: * An applicant must have been awarded the highest care component of DLA before an application can be accepted.

The 93 Fund makes cash payments which may be used to employ one or more assistants for personal and domestic care. Nursing care, childcare costs, costs of equipment and respite care in a residential or nursing home cannot be covered. The money may not be used to employ a close relative living in the same house.

The Fund makes a financial assessment of an applicant's ability to contribute to their care costs and the following would be regarded as available:

- half of the care component of their Disability Living Allowance;

- all of their Severe Disability Premium (if paid with Income Support);

- all of their Special Transitional Allowance (if paid with Income Support);

- all income above Income Support level (when applicant is not on Income Support).

Appendix B: Details of disabled people referred to in the report

Name[a]	Age range	Household	Disability	Funding[b]	Type of assistance[c]
Ahmed	36-40	Spouse	Muscular dystrophy	LA & ILF 93 Fund	Brokerage/2 PAs
Anna	56-60	Alone	Multiple sclerosis	LA	LA Homecare & brokerage/1 PA
Barbara	51-55	2 children	Osteo-arthritis	LA & ILF 93 Fund	Brokerage/1 PA
Beth	41-45	Residential care	Multiple sclerosis	DSS	
Brian	41-45	Alone	Cerebral palsy	LA	CSVs
Caroline	31-35	Alone	Friedreich's ataxia	LA & ILF Ext Fund	Agency
Christine	56-60	Spouse	Stroke	LA & HA	LA Homecare & agency
Dan	41-45	Alone	Spinal injury	LA, HA &ILF 93 Fund	Direct payments/8 PAs
Dave	31-35	Mother & brother	Spinal injury	LA	Agency
Dora	46-50	Alone	Osteo-arthritis	LA & ILF 93 Fund	Brokerage/1 PA
Doreen	21-25	Alone	Spinal injury	LA & ILF 93 Fund	Direct payments/3 PAs
Elisabeth	46-50	Alone	Motor neurone damage	LA, HA & ILF 93 Fund	Agency
Frances	36-40	Alone	Spinal injury	LA & ILF Ext Fund	Agency & 1 PA
Gillian	41-45	Spouse	Cerebral palsy	LA & ILF 93 Fund	Brokerage/2 PAs
Helen	36-40	Alone	Spinal injury	LA & ILF 93 Fund	Agency & 1 PA
Hilary	36-40	2 children	Multiple sclerosis & stroke	LA & ILF 93 Fund	Direct payments 4 PAs
Ian	46-50	Spouse & child	Parkinson's disease	LA & ILF 93 Fund	Agency

Name[a]	Age range	Household	Disability	Funding[b]	Type of assistance[c]
Jane	61-65	Spouse	Spinal injury & kidney failure	LA & ILF Ext Fund	Direct payments 2 PAs
Jacqueline	41-45	Spouse	Multiple sclerosis	LA	Agency
Jenny	51-55	Alone	Spinal injury	LA & ILF 93 Fund	LA Homecare & agency
Jim	26-30	Parents	Head injury	LA & ILF Ext Fund	LA Homecare & agency
Joe	56-60	Spouse	Alzheimers	LA & ILF 93 Fund	Agency
Julie	31-35	Alone	Tetraplegia	LA & ILF Ext Fund	Direct payments/3 PAs
Ken	61-65	Spouse	Spinal injury	LA & ILF 93 Fund	Brokerage/1 PA
Kirsten	41-45	Spouse & children	Multiple sclerosis	LA	Agency
Laura	31-35	Alone	Spinal injury	LA & ILF 93 Fund	Agency & 1 PA
Len	21-25	Mother	Cerebral palsy	LA & ILF Ext Fund	LA Homecare & agencies
Margaret	41-45	Alone	Spinal injury	LA & ILF 93 Fund	Brokerage/1 PAs
Mark	36-40	Alone	Spinal injury	LA	Agency
Martha	66-70	Alone	Arthritis & stroke	LA & ILF Ext Fund	Agency
Mary	36-40	Alone	Multiple sclerosis	LA	Agency
Mike	41-45	Alone	Heart disease & stroke	LA & ILF 93 Fund	Agency & PAs
Mohammed	41-45	Alone	Multiple sclerosis	LA & ILF 93 Fund	Agency
Nora	46-50	Spouse	Polio	LA & ILF 93 Fund	Brokerage/1 PA
Parveen	26-30	Parents	Arthrogryophosis	LA	Agency
Pat	46-50	Alone	Multiple sclerosis & osteo-arthritis	LA	Brokerage/2 PAs

Name[a]	Age range	Household	Disability	Funding[b]	Type of assistance[c]
Pauline	51-55	Alone	Multiple sclerosis	LA	Agency
Richard	21-25	Parents	Friedreich's ataxia	LA & ILF 93 Fund	Agency
Robert	31-35	Mother	Multiple sclerosis	LA & ILF Ext Fund	Agencies
Samantha	51-55	Alone	Spinal injury	LA & ILF Ext Fund	Brokerage/5 PAs
Sarah	36-40	Spouse & 3 children	Multiple sclerosis	LA & ILF 93 Fund	Brokerage/2 PAs
Simon	26-30	Alone	Spinal injury	LA & HA	Agencies
Sue	41-45	Alone	Multiple sclerosis	LA & ILF 93 Fund	Direct payments/agency
Tracey	36-40	Alone	Cerebral palsy	LA	Agency
Wendy	36-40	Residential care	Brain tumour	LA & HA	
William	51-55	Spouse	Rheumatoid arthritis	LA & ILF 93 Fund	Agency

Notes:
[a] not the person's real name
[b] excluding direct health service provision
[c] brokerage = LA indirect payments; PA = personal assistant employed with LA (in)direct payments and/or ILF award